Biopreparedness and Public Health

NATO Science for Peace and Security Series

This Series presents the results of scientific meetings supported under the NATO Programme: Science for Peace and Security (SPS).

The NATO SPS Programme supports meetings in the following Key Priority areas: (1) Defence Against Terrorism; (2) Countering other Threats to Security and (3) NATO, Partner and Mediterranean Dialogue Country Priorities. The types of meeting supported are generally "Advanced Study Institutes" and "Advanced Research Workshops". The NATO SPS Series collects together the results of these meetings. The meetings are co-organized by scientists from NATO countries and scientists from NATO's "Partner" or "Mediterranean Dialogue" countries. The observations and recommendations made at the meetings, as well as the contents of the volumes in the Series, reflect those of participants and contributors only; they should not necessarily be regarded as reflecting NATO views or policy.

Advanced Study Institutes (ASI) are high-level tutorial courses to convey the latest developments in a subject to an advanced-level audience

Advanced Research Workshops (ARW) are expert meetings where an intense but informal exchange of views at the frontiers of a subject aims at identifying directions for future action

Following a transformation of the programme in 2006 the Series has been re-named and re-organised. Recent volumes on topics not related to security, which result from meetings supported under the programme earlier, may be found in the NATO Science Series.

The Series is published by IOS Press, Amsterdam, and Springer, Dordrecht, in conjunction with the NATO Emerging Security Challenges Division.

Sub-Series

A.	Chemistry and Biology	Springer
B.	Physics and Biophysics	Springer
C.	Environmental Security	Springer
D.	Information and Communication Security	IOS Press
E.	Human and Societal Dynamics	IOS Press

http://www.nato.int/science
http://www.springer.com
http://www.iospress.nl

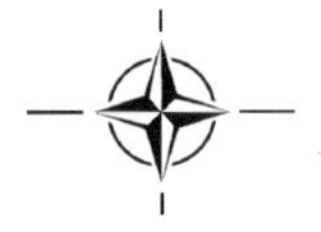

Series A: Chemistry and Biology

Biopreparedness and Public Health

Exploring Synergies

edited by

Iris Hunger
Carl Friedrich von Weizsäcker Centre for Science and Peace Research
University of Hamburg, Hamburg, Germany

Vladan Radosavljevic
Military Academy, University of Defence, Belgrade, Serbia

Goran Belojevic
Institute of Hygiene and Medical Ecology, Faculty of Medicine
University of Belgrade, Serbia

and

Lisa D. Rotz
Centers for Disease Control and Prevention, Atlanta, Georgia, USA

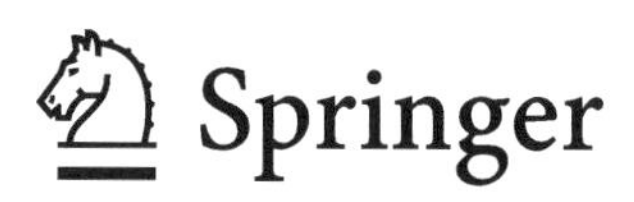

Published in Cooperation with NATO Emerging Security Challenges Division

Results from the NATO Advanced Research Workshop on
Exploring Synergies between Bioterrorism Preparedness and General Public
Health Measures
Belgrade, Serbia
15–17 November, 2010

Library of Congress Control Number: 2012944988

ISBN 978-94-007-5299-3 (PB)
ISBN 978-94-007-5272-6 (HB)
ISBN 978-94-007-5273-3 (e-book)
DOI 10.1007/978-94-007-5273-3

Published by Springer,
P.O. Box 17, 3300 AA Dordrecht, The Netherlands

www.springer.com

Printed on acid-free paper

Preface

The threat from the terrorist use of pathogens has been a major security concern in recent years, particularly after the anthrax letter attacks in the USA in 2001. This threat of intentional outbreaks of diseases stands side by side with the constantly changing natural threat from diseases, epidemics, and pandemics, as illustrated in recent years by the H1N1 influenza pandemic, the SARS outbreak, and the H5N1 avian influenza event. While naturally occurring diseases – both newly emerging and well-known ones – claim the life and health of many people year after year, bioterrorism events have so far had a very limited health impact.

Protection, prevention, and response measures for natural disease outbreaks and for bioterrorism events differ greatly between countries. At the national level these aspects all too often are handled by different actors with different approaches under different funding arrangements. In many states, resources and political attention are so stretched that the bioterrorism threat is not dealt with at all. While natural and deliberate outbreaks of disease differ in a number of ways – e.g., the types of diseases involved, risk communications, or the legal follow-up – in many areas the differences are likely to be small, in particular those involving non-disease-specific public health detection and response activities. Finding these areas of overlap, identifying the differences and the gaps in preparedness measures, and thereby contributing to streamlining response measures so as to enable them to protect public health from all three types of biological threats – natural, accidental, deliberate – is an urgent need for countries worldwide, and in particular for countries whose public health systems are already overburdened by natural disease response.

To address the issue, 34 experts from 17 European countries, including Turkey, as well as the USA, Israel, the World Health Organization, and the European Centre for Disease Prevention and Control gathered for a NATO-sponsored Advanced Research Workshop entitled "Exploring synergies between bioterrorism preparedness and general public health measures" in the Serbian Academy of Sciences and Arts (SANU) in Belgrade, Serbia, during 15–17 November 2010. In addition to the 34 workshop participants, the first half-day of the workshop, with introductory and more general presentations, drew a number of local experts, illustrating the interest in the issues under discussion. Most notably, the workshop participants welcomed Zoran Jeftic, State Secretary from the Serbian Ministry of Defence, and Lee Litzenberger, Deputy Head of Mission of the US Embassy in Belgrade, who addressed the gathering during the opening ceremony.

The workshop focused on Southeastern Europe, a region where some of the diseases caused by agents of bioterrorism concern, such as tularemia or certain types of hemorrhagic fevers, are endemic. This region also regularly experiences natural outbreaks of other diseases whose causative agents also have relevance as potential bioweapons risk agents. The workshop was not only an opportunity to learn from local experiences in fighting these diseases, but also a unique occasion for regional and global networking.

The workshop addressed the current level of threat from naturally occurring infectious diseases and the current bioterrorism threat, the response and preparedness efforts in different countries of Southeastern Europe, France, Germany, Israel, Poland, the United States, the European Union, and globally. From these empirical data, commonalities, differences, and gaps among states' efforts and between general public health measures and biopreparedness were extracted and discussed. Lessons were derived on where bioterrorism preparedness and response measures at the moment and in the future can benefit other areas of public health and vice versa.

To capture the information that was exchanged during the workshop and further explore synergies for public health preparedness, selected workshop participants were asked to write detailed case studies on the relationship between biopreparedness efforts and other public health measures in their countries or their international organizations, which – together with a number of chapters on more general bio-threat related topics – are assembled in this international scientific monograph.

The thanks of the editors of this volume go to NATO's Science for Peace and Security Programme for funding the original workshop, to the Serbian Academy of Sciences and Arts (SANU) – and in particular to Academician Prof. Ljubisav Rakic – for hosting the workshop in Belgrade, and to two external reviewers who contributed valuable comments during the preparation of this book – Brig. Gen. (ret) Mario Stefano Peragallo, MD, Consultant in Preventive Medicine and Hygiene, Italian Army Medical Research Center, Rome (Italy), and Brig. Gen. (ret) Ioannis Galatas, MD, Consultant in Allergy and Clinical Immunology, Medical/Hospital CBRNE Planner, and Senior Asymmetric Threats Analyst, Athens (Greece).

Last but not least, the editors thank the participants and guests at the workshop, and all the authors of this book who were willing to give part of their limited time and share their experiences to make further advancements on the route towards a world free from the threat of deliberate disease.

December 2011 Atlanta, Belgrade and Hamburg

Iris Hunger
University of Hamburg
Hamburg, Germany

Goran Belojevic
University of Belgrade
Belgrade, Serbia

Vladan Radosavljevic
Military Academy, University of Defence
Belgrade, Serbia

Lisa Rotz
Centers for Disease Control and Prevention
Atlanta, USA

Contents

Chapter 1
Introduction

Iris Hunger

Abstract Health and security have become intertwined in recent years. While this has been welcomed by many experts because it led to an increase in funding for selected public health activities, others worry that this development will distract from sustaining and improving basic public health services. The challenge, in particular in low- and mid-income countries, is to improve the public health system as a whole and simultaneously provide an appropriate level of awareness and response capability for the low-likelihood, but high-consequence event of a bioterrorist attack.

1.1 Connecting Health and Security

For a long time, public health was an issue which security experts did not care about. Over the last decade, this has changed. Epidemics, gaps in disease surveillance, and lack of public health intervention capacities are increasingly perceived as a threat to national security, regional stability and international peace. Starting in the late 1990s, health has more and more been conceived as a security issue.

This re-conceptualization of health as a security issue started in a number of think tanks that described infectious diseases – in particular the HIV/AIDS pandemic – as a threat to peace and security. Promoting health globally, it was postulated, is not just a matter of "doing good", but also a critical aspect of foreign policy and national security [6–8]. Already in April 2000, U.S. President Bill Clinton announced that AIDS would be treated as a threat to U.S. national security. And in July 2000, the

I. Hunger (✉)
Research Group for Biological Arms Control, Carl Friedrich von Weizsäcker
Centre for Science and Peace Research, University of Hamburg,
Beim Schlump 83, 20144 Hamburg, Germany
e-mail: irishunger@versanet.de

I. Hunger et al. (eds.), *Biopreparedness and Public Health: Exploring Synergies*,
NATO Science for Peace and Security Series A: Chemistry and Biology,
DOI 10.1007/978-94-007-5273-3_1,

United Nations Security Council passed Resolution 1308, which declared that action was necessary before the AIDS pandemic could further threaten world stability ([10]: 30).

The World Health Organization (WHO) initially rejected a formal relationship between health and security. There was the fear that neutral health work could be misused for political goals. It was not before 2007, that "global public health security"entered the vocabulary of WHO [13].

Meanwhile, arms control and non-proliferation experts dealing with biological weapons issues increasingly turned their attention away from verifying compliance with the global bioweapons ban and towards countering bioterrorism and securing public health. During the past decade, disease surveillance has been one of the few issues that states parties to the 1972 Biological Weapons Convention have been discussing during their annual consultations in Geneva [1].

There is a question in many experts' minds to what degree security and health can be and should (or should not) be connected and how best to link the two. For many it is a positive development that public health – local and global – is receiving attention from the security community, because that attention has led to substantial additional funding. Money for health is always a good thing, independent of source and motivation, the argument goes. But there is also some uneasiness about the fact that health has been turned into a security issue in the last 10 years. There is concern that global health is transformed from a humanitarian issue into an issue of national interest, which could lead to shaping the international health agenda more narrowly around the diseases that are of security concern to Western donor countries [4]. WHO noted in one of its recent annual reports that primary public health care (such as the nurse visiting a village once a month) does not get the attention needed for sustainable health improvements [14].

1.2 The Mismatch Between Public Health and Biodefence Funding

The threat from the terrorist use of diseases has received much attention in recent years, particularly after the anthrax letter attacks in the USA in 2001. This threat of intentionally-caused outbreaks of diseases has joined the long-existing and constantly changing natural threat from diseases, epidemics, and pandemics. While the disease burden from naturally occurring diseases continues to be heavy, bioterrorism – fortunately – has remained a largely hypothetical threat.

Looking at the resources available to counter both threats, a glaring mismatch is evident between the number of death and illness from natural disease outbreaks compared to the ones caused by bioterrorism on the one hand, and the funding available to prepare for such events on the other. Illustrative examples are listed in Table 1.1.

While the impact of naturally occurring infectious diseases is to a certain degree foreseeable and a lot of experience with preventing, limiting, countering, responding to, and recovering from natural disease outbreaks exists, bioterrorism events have

Table 1.1 Illustrative quotes and numbers on the mismatch between disease burden and funding of countermeasure development from natural public health threats and bioterrorism

Disease burden	Countermeasure development
Estimated 1.7 million people died from tuberculosis in 2009 [15]	"Funding for [tuberculosis] control continues to increase and will reach almost US$5 billion in 2011. … Compared with the funding requirements estimated in the Global Plan [to Stop TB], the funding gap is approximately US$ 1 billion in 2011. Given the scale-up of interventions set out in the plan, this could increase to US$3 billion by 2015 without intensified efforts to mobilize more resources" [15]
Estimated 781,000 people died from malaria in 2009 [16]	"International funding for malaria control has risen steeply in the past decade. Disbursements reached their highest ever levels in 2009 at US$ 1.5 billion, but new commitments for malaria control appear to have stagnated in 2010, at US$ 1.8 billion.… The amounts committed to malaria, while substantial, still fall short of the resources required for malaria control, estimated at more than US$ 6 billion for the year 2010" [16]
Estimated 1.8 million people died from AIDS-related illnesses in 2009 [12]	"A total of US$ 15.9 billion was available for the AIDS response in 2009, US$10 billion short of what is needed in 2010" [12]
Five people have been killed in bioterrorist attacks since 1900 [9, 11]	Biodefence spending in the United States has grown from USD 0.6 billion in 2001 to USD 8.1 billion in 2005. USD 6.5 billion were budgeted for 2011 [3]
	Biodefence and biosecurity activities and funding have increased in many – mostly Western – countries around the world. [3, 5] Cooperative projects on biosecurity are funded in a number of non-Western states. (See, for example, [2].)

been so rare that knowledge is largely hypothetical. Undoubtedly, bioterrorist attacks have the potential to be unexpected mass casualty events. How likely such events are, how exactly they would look like, and how best to respond remains very much debated. The uncertainty associated with the bioterrorism threat makes public health preparedness planning for such events practically and politically very difficult.

1.3 Aim and Structure of This Book

In a world of limited financial resources states can ill afford to create parallel structures for preventing and preparing for natural disease events and for human-made, deliberately caused disease outbreaks. While there are obviously a number of differences between natural and deliberate outbreaks of disease – e.g. the types of diseases involved, the extent of decontamination necessary, or the legal follow-up – there also are large areas where differences are likely to be small, in particular in the areas of detection (e.g. through disease surveillance) and non-disease-specific public health responses. After all, in both cases one deals with a disease outbreak.

At the moment, preparedness for natural disease outbreaks and bioterrorism preparedness are all too often dealt with by different actors with different approaches under different funding arrangements. Describing and comparing the existing relationships between measures to protect public health in general and measures to prepare for the unlikely but potentially catastrophic event of a bioterrorism attack, and drawing lessons for optimizing this relationship is the aim of this book.

The book focuses on countries in southeastern Europe, a region where some of the diseases caused by agents of bioterrorism concern are endemic, such as tularemia or Crimean Congo hemorrhagic fever. This region suffers regularly from natural outbreaks of bioweapons-relevant diseases. To allow a broader comparative analysis, case studies on a number of countries from outside this region are also included.

The book is divided in two parts. In the first part, the scene is set. Jonathan Tucker, a policy analyst on chemical and biological security issues, Washington, DC (USA), assesses the current bioweapons threat. Vladan Radosavljevic from the Military Academy, University of Defence, Belgrade (Serbia), offers a framework for differentiating between a biological attack and other epidemics. The differences in responding to natural and unnatural disease outbreaks are analysed by Amesh Adalja from the Center for Biosecurity, University of Pittsburgh Medical Center, Baltimore (USA).

The following three chapters address selected public health issues from a supranational perspective. Catherine Smallwood and colleagues from Health Security and Environment, World Health Organization, Geneva (Switzerland) offer WHO's perspective on managing acute public health events. Dorit Nitzan Kaluski, WHO Country Office Serbia, Belgrade (Serbia), and Maria Ruseva, WHO Regional Office for Europe, Copenhagen (Denmark), describe the recent reforms of public health systems in countries in the South-eastern Europe Health Network. And Massimo Ciotti, European Centre for Disease Prevention and Control, Stockholm (Sweden), portrays health security and disease detection efforts in the European Union.

The second part of the book contains case studies on individual countries with a focus on countries from southeastern Europe. Authors of the country studies were asked to address the following questions:

- What are the main public health threats (in terms of infectious diseases) in your country? How important does your country perceive bioterrorism as a potential threat?
- How is preparedness and response to health emergencies organized in your country? How does preparedness and response to a bioterrorism event differ in your country from preparedness and response to other health emergencies?
- What role does the military, in contrast to civilian agencies, play in preparedness and response to natural and human-made health emergencies?

The country case studies cover:

- Bulgaria, authored by Raynichka Mihaylova-Garnizova and Kamen Plochev, Military Medical Academy, Clinic of Infectious Diseases, Sofia (Bulgaria);
- France, authored by Elisande Nexon, Fondation pour la recherche stratégique, Paris (France);

- Germany, authored by Christine Uhlenhaut and Lars Schaade, Robert Koch Institute, Berlin (Germany), and Ernst-Jürgen Finke, scientific consultant in medical biological defence, Munich (Germany);
- Greece, authored by Nikolaos Zaras, Special Joint CBRN Company, Hellenic Army, Athens (Greece);
- Israel, authored by Adini Bruria and Daniel Laor, Emergency and Disaster Management Division, Ministry of Health, Tel Aviv (Israel), and Manfred Green, School of Public Health, University of Haifa, Haifa (Israel);
- Italy, authored by Francesco Urbano, Italian Army Logistic Branch, Medical Department, Rome (Italy), and Maria Rita Gismondo, Faculty of Medicine and Surgery, "Luigi Sacco" University Hospital, Milan (Italy);
- Poland, authored by Anna Bielecka and Janusz Kocik, Military Institute of Hygiene and Epidemiology, Department of Epidemiology, Warsaw (Poland);
- Romania, authored by Alexandru Rafila and Daniela Pitigoi, University of Medicine and Pharmacy "Carol Davila" and National Institute for Infectious Diseases "Prof. Dr. Matei Bals", Bucharest (Romania);
- Serbia, authored by Goran Belojevic, Institute of Hygiene and Medical Ecology, Faculty of Medicine, University of Belgrade, Belgrade (Serbia);
- Turkey, authored by Gurkan Mert, Gulhane Military Medical Academy, Ankara (Turkey); and
- USA, authored by Lisa Rotz, Centers for Disease Control and Prevention (CDC), Atlanta, GA (USA), and Marcelle Layton, New York City Department of Health and Mental Hygiene, New York, NY (USA).

In their concluding remarks, the editors provide a summary and comparison of public health preparedness efforts for natural and unnatural disease outbreaks in the countries covered by the case studies, and offer recommendations on the relationship between biopreparedness and wider public health.

The editors were very sorry to learn about the death of Jonathan Tucker during the preparation of the book manuscript. Jonathan Tucker died unexpectedly in July 2011. He was an internationally esteemed expert on chemical and biological weapons, arms control and non-proliferation, on security aspects of biotechnologies, on dangerous infectious diseases, and on unconventional terrorism. He worked at the interface of science and policy in very different institutions including the US Congressional Office of Technology Assessment, the US Arms Control and Disarmament Agency, the Center for Non-Proliferation Studies, and the Federation of American Scientists. Jonathan Tucker was highly respected for his balanced, careful research, and enormous productivity. The world is a safer place because of his work. His many friends and colleagues around the world feel his loss sorely.

References

1. Bansak KC (2011) Enhancing compliance with an evolving treaty: a task for an improved BWC intersessional process. Arms Control Today 41. http://www.armscontrol.org/act/2011_06/Bansak. Accessed 14 Sep 2011
2. BEP (2011) Biosecurity engagement project. US Department of State. http://www.bepstate.net/index.html. Accessed 14 Sep 2011
3. BWPP (2011) Bioweapons monitor. Country report USA. http://www.bwpp.org/ documents/BWM%202011%20WEB.pdf. Accessed 21 Dec 2011
4. Elbe S (2008) Securitizing epidemics: three lessons from history. Paper presented at "Impacting health, the environment and global governance. The challenges of taking a security approach". International seminar organized by the Institut Francais des Relations Internationales (IFRI). Paris. September 2008. www.stefanelbe.com/6.html. Accessed 21 Dec 2011
5. Hunger I (2005) Confidence building needs transparency: a summary of data submitted under the bioweapons convention's confidence building measures 1987–2003. The Sunshine Project. http://www.biological-arms-control.org/publications/hunger_CBM.pdf. Accessed 20 Dec 2011
6. Hunter RE, Anthony CR, Lurie N (2002) Make world health the new Marshall Plan. RAND Rev 26(2). http://www.rand.org/publications/ randreview/issues/rr-08-02/worldhealth.html. Accessed 18 Dec 2011
7. ICG (2001) HIV/AIDS as a security issue. Issues report no.1. International Crisis Group. http://www.crisisgroup.org/en/regions/africa/001-hiv-aids-as-a-security-issue.aspx. Accessed 20 Dec 2011
8. Lee K, McInnes C (2003) Health, foreign policy and security: a discussion paper. UK Global Health Programme working paper no.1. The Nuffield Trust. London. http://www.nuffieldtrust.org.uk/sites/files/nuffield/publication/health-foreign-policy-and-security-apr03.pdf. Accessed 17 Dec 2011
9. Leitenberg M (2005) Assessing the biological weapons and bioterrorism threat. Strategic Studies Institute. United States Army War College: Carlisle, Pennsylvania. http://www.strategicstudiesinstitute.army.mil/pdffiles/pub639.pdf. Accessed 21 Dec 2011
10. Sheehan CC (2008) Securitizing the HIV/AIDS pandemic in U.S. foreign policy. Dissertation. The American University. http://books.google.de/books?id=WuLE5jBS0esC&printsec=frontcover&hl=de&source=gbs_ge_summary_r&cad=0#v=onepage&q&f=false. Accessed 24 Sep 2011
11. Tucker JB, Sands A (1999) An unlikely threat. Bull At Sci 55(4):46–52
12. UNAIDS (2010) Report on the global AIDS epidemic. http://www.unaids.org/ globalreport/documents/20101123_GlobalReport_full_en.pdf. Accessed 24 Sep 2011
13. WHO (2007) The world health report 2007. A safer future: global public health security in the 21st century. http://www.who.int/whr/2007/whr07_en.pdf. Accessed 24 Sep 2011
14. WHO (2008) The world health report. Primary health care now more than ever. http://www.who.int/whr/2008/whr08_en.pdf. Accessed 20 Dec 2011
15. WHO (2010a) Global tuberculosis control. Summary. http://whqlibdoc.who.int/ publications/2010/9789241564069_eng.pdf. Accessed 24 Sep 2011
16. WHO (2010b) World malaria report. Executive summary. http://www.who.int/malaria/world_malaria_report_2010/malaria2010_summary_keypoints_en.pdf. Accessed 24 Sep 2011

Chapter 2
The Current Bioweapons Threat

Jonathan B. Tucker†

Abstract According to unclassified U.S. government sources, states of biological weapons (BW) proliferation concern include China, Iran, North Korea, Russia, and Syria. Assessing the BW threat is challenging, however, because illicit development and production can be concealed at dual-use industrial sites such as vaccine plants, and only tens of kilograms of an agent like dried anthrax spores can be militarily significant. The lack of unambiguous technical signatures of BW-related activity means that most estimates of foreign capabilities draw heavily on human intelligence sources, yet spies and defectors are notoriously unreliable. A key factor driving BW proliferation is the perceived military utility of biological weapons, which may include strategic deterrence, asymmetric warfare, or covert operations. Globalization of the biotechnology industry has expanded trade in dual-use materials and production equipment, increasing the risks of diversion and misuse for BW purposes. With the advent of flexible biological manufacturing systems, it has also become possible for countries to acquire a "latent" capacity for BW production during a crisis or war. Since the 2001 anthrax letter attacks, sub-state actors have become a prominent part of the threat matrix, but terrorist acquisition and use of BW requires both the motivation to use disease as a weapon and the technical capability to do so, a combination that is quite rare. At present the threat of mass-casualty BW attacks emanates primarily from nation-states, while terrorist use of biological weapons will likely remain limited in scale and impact. Nevertheless, the emergence of new biotechnologies with a potential for misuse could result in more damaging incidents of bioterrorism in the future.

The editors mourn the loss of Dr. Jonathan B. Tucker, who died unexpectedly during the preparation of this book.

J.B. Tucker† (Deceased)

I. Hunger et al. (eds.), *Biopreparedness and Public Health: Exploring Synergies*, NATO Science for Peace and Security Series A: Chemistry and Biology,
DOI 10.1007/978-94-007-5273-3_2,

2.1 Introduction

A starting point for assessing the current threat of biological weapons (BW) is the unclassified arms control compliance report prepared periodically by the U.S. State Department, most recently in July 2010, although it does not cover all countries of proliferation concern. The section of the report addressing compliance with the 1972 Biological and Toxin Weapons Convention (BWC) suggests that Iran, North Korea, and Syria (a signatory state) may have active BW programmes and that China and Russia have been less than forthcoming about their past offensive activities [16, pp. 10–26].

Because the BWC lacks any formal multilateral verification mechanisms, these assessments are based on U.S. national intelligence capabilities. The 2010 State Department report uses extremely hedged language, however, suggesting the high level of uncertainty that surrounds the BWC compliance of several countries. The entry on Iran, for example, reads: "Available information indicates that Iran has remained engaged in dual-use BW-related activities. The United States notes that Iran may not have ended activities prohibited by the BWC, although available information does not conclusively indicate that Iran is currently conducting activities prohibited by the Convention" [16, p. 16].

This uncertainty stems from the fact that monitoring clandestine BW programmes is a challenging task for several reasons. First, BW development and production capabilities can be concealed at ostensibly legitimate industrial sites, such as vaccine plants or facilities for the production of single-cell protein or biopesticide. Second, the equipment and know-how needed for the manufacture of BW agents is entirely dual-use, although technologies for weaponization and delivery are more specialized. Third, because only tens of kilograms of an agent such as dried anthrax spores can be militarily significant, even small-scale production facilities are relevant from a security standpoint. Fourth, proliferant states often use deception and denial techniques to conceal their BW-related activities, as was demonstrated by the cat-and-mouse game played by Iraq and United Nations biological weapons inspectors after the 1991 Persian Gulf War. Finally, since the terrorist attacks in the United States on September 11, 2001, and the subsequent mailing of letters contaminated with anthrax bacterial spores, the biodefence programmes of several countries have expanded dramatically, providing a potential cover for offensive BW development.

Because of the difficulty of monitoring clandestine BW programmes, several countries have violated the BWC in the past with impunity, including the Soviet Union, apartheid South Africa, and Saddam Hussein's Iraq. From the 1970s through the early 1990s, Moscow conducted a vast, top-secret biological warfare programme that was partially concealed inside a pharmaceutical development and production complex known as Biopreparat. The full scale and scope of this effort were not detected by Western intelligence agencies at the time and were only revealed after the defection of high-level Biopreparat officials in the late 1980s and early 1990s [1].

The lack of clear technical signatures of biological weapons development and production means that most current estimates of foreign BW capabilities draw heavily on human sources. Unfortunately, spies and defectors are notoriously unreliable. Before the 2003 Iraq War, for example, the CIA was seriously misled by an Iraqi source code-named "Curveball," who claimed that after the UN weapons inspectors the country in December 1998, the regime of Saddam Hussein had reconstituted its BW programme by deploying mobile biological production facilities. The CIA unwisely placed credence in this uncorroborated source, who later turned out to have fabricated his story out of whole cloth [4]. In sum, for the reasons noted above, publicly available lists of countries suspected of possessing or seeking biological weapons should be viewed as little more than educated guesses.

2.2 Perceived Military Utility

An important factor affecting the state-level BW threat is the perceived military utility of biological weapons. Most of the microbial pathogens that states have developed in the past as BW agents are zoonotic bacteria and viruses that infect humans as well as animals but are not transmissible from person to person; examples include the causative agents of anthrax, tularemia, Q fever, and Venezuelan equine encephalitis. Such non-contagious agents are best suited for targeted military use because only troops directly exposed to the agent cloud would be affected. During the Cold War, however, the Soviet Union developed two contagious agents (the smallpox virus and the plague bacterium) as strategic biological weapons for attacks on U.S. cities. Soviet military planners apparently assumed that the delivery of these agents against distant targets in the United States would trigger local epidemics that would not spread widely enough to boomerang against the Soviet population [1].

Because microbial BW agents have an asymptomatic incubation period lasting days or even weeks after infection before they produce incapacitating symptoms, they have little tactical utility on the battlefield. Instead, paramilitary or special-operations forces might employ biological weapons for non-time-sensitive operations, such as attacking troop reinforcements or command-and-control centers deep behind enemy lines or targeting dug-in troops or insurgents in remote areas or mountain redoubts. Anti-crop or anti-livestock agents might also be used for covert sabotage attacks in order to undermine the agricultural economy of an adversary nation.

Some countries that are currently assessed to possess a BW capability appear to view it as a means of holding a potential adversary's populated urban centers at risk for deterrence purposes. Syrian President Bashar al-Assad, for example, once suggested obliquely in an interview that his country was justified in acquiring biological and chemical weapons as a means of balancing Israel's undeclared nuclear weapons capability. "We are a country which is [partly] occupied and from time to time we are exposed to Israeli aggression," Assad said. "It is natural for us to look for means to defend ourselves. It is not difficult to get most of these weapons anywhere in the world and they can be obtained at any time" [2].

Acquiring a BW capability may also be attractive to militarily weak states as an asymmetrical means of deterring or countering conventional attack by a much stronger military power. Before the 1991 Persian Gulf War, for example, Iraqi leader Saddam Hussein ordered the crash production of a stockpile of biological weapons, including aerial bombs and missile warheads filled with anthrax spores, botulinum toxin, and aflatoxin. Saddam viewed this BW capability as an "ace in the hole" to secure his regime from the internal and external opponents seeking to topple him from power. Although it is not clear how a secret weapons programme could serve as an effective deterrent against the United States and Israel, Saddam may have counted on the rumors before the Gulf War that he possessed biological weapons [9].

After Iraq's military defeat, Saddam ordered the unilateral destruction of the biological weapons stocks so they would not be found by UN inspectors. At the same time, however, he continued to maintain ambiguity about whether or not the weapons still existed in order to deter Iran as well as his domestic enemies, the Shiites and the Kurds. The CIA's Iraq Survey Group, which searched in vain for Iraq's suspected weapons of mass destruction in the aftermath of the 2003 Iraq War, concluded that Saddam had bluffed about possessing biological and chemical weapons because he felt vulnerable without them [7].

2.3 Impact of Economic Globalization

In recent decades, economic globalization has affected the dynamics of BW proliferation. Several developing countries, including China, Cuba, India, Malaysia, and Singapore, have invested heavily in industrial microbiology as a vehicle for economic development. The global spread of the biotechnology industry has complicated the task of regulating the international trade in items of biological production equipment, such as fermenters and spray-driers, increasing the risk of their diversion and misuse for bioweapons production. Despite the existence of the Australia Group, an informal forum of more than 40 countries that harmonize their national export controls on dual-use materials and equipment relevant to chemical and biological weapons, suppliers in countries that do not participate in the Australia Group (such as China, Cuba, India, and Russia) have sold dual-use items to countries of BW proliferation concern.

Another troubling development is what has been called "latent" or "virtual" BW proliferation. With the advent of flexible biological manufacturing systems that can switch rapidly from one product to another in response to shifts in market demand, dedicated factories are no longer required for the production of BW agents. Instead, it has become possible for countries to acquire and maintain a standby mobilization capacity for biological weapons production at dual-use facilities without overtly violating the BWC. A would-be cheater could perform the research, development, and testing for an offensive BW programme in secret and then maintain a latent production capacity in distributed form at several locations until a political decision was made to break out of the BWC and acquire a weapons stockpile. At that time, key items of dual-use equipment, and the technical teams needed to operate them, could be brought together to initiate a BW production campaign. The short period—measured in weeks—required to manufacture a militarily significant stockpile might prevent an adversary from bolstering its medical defenses in a timely manner.

Mobilization programmes at dual-use biological facilities are very hard to detect, even with intrusive on-site inspections such as those conducted by the UN weapons inspectors in Iraq. Accordingly, evidence that a state has acquired a breakout BW production capability would depend on intelligence about the intentions of the country's leaders. The high-placed human sources needed to collect such information, however, are difficult to recruit. Latent proliferation also poses a major challenge for biological arms control. Because the BWC compliance of a dual-use production facility is largely a matter of intent, a state party would violate the treaty only when it started to produce biological agents "of types and in quantities that have no justification for prophylactic, protective or other peaceful purposes." Given the difficulty of monitoring illicit production, it is far from certain that such a violation would be detected.

2.4 Non-state Actors

Since the mailing in autumn 2001 of letters contaminated with anthrax bacterial spores, killing five people in the United States and infecting 17 others, non-state actors have become a prominent part of the BW threat matrix. Compared to states, terrorist organizations are hard to deter and thus have fewer constraints on the use of biological weapons, although their technical capabilities tend to be significantly lower.

To acquire a BW capability, a terrorist group must be motivated to employ infectious disease as a weapon and must also possess the necessary technical resources. On the motivational side, only a small number of terrorist organizations have sought biological weapons in the past, for several reasons. First, terrorist groups tend to be conservative in their choice of weapons and tactics, innovating only when forced to do so, and they typically select materials and delivery systems that are readily available and have predictable effects, such as high explosives. Second, politically motivated terrorist organizations (such as the Irish Republican Army) have not pursued biological weapons because their use would be perceived as disproportionate and illegitimate, alienating the group's supporters and potential recruits and provoking a severe crackdown by government authorities. Third, the uncertainties associated with the effective use of biological agents are considerable, raising doubts in the minds of the potential perpetrators about whether or not a planned attack will be successful [10].

The types of terrorist organizations most likely to pursue biological weapons are those with an extreme religious or ideological worldview, such as apocalyptic cults, white supremacists, and jihadist organizations. Such groups are more inclined than more traditional, politically motivated terrorist organizations to inflict indiscriminate casualties and to pursue risky, innovative tactics. Al-Qaeda, for example, launched a BW programme code-named Al Zabadi (the Arabic word for "yogurt") in May 1999 with an initial investment of a few thousand dollars. At training camps in Afghanistan, Al-Qaeda operatives established makeshift labs where they experimented with the plant toxin ricin (suitable for assassination purposes) and attempted unsuccessfully on at least two occasions to acquire a virulent strain of anthrax [13].

Beyond the motivation to acquire and use biological weapons, would-be bioterrorists must possess the specialized know-how and financial resources needed to acquire, weaponize, and deliver highly infectious and lethal agents. Popular accounts in the news media generally underestimate the technical hurdles involved in acquiring biological weapons and delivering them effectively. To develop an anthrax weapon, for example, would-be bioterrorists would have to obtain and cultivate a virulent strain of the bacterium, induce it to sporulate, process the spores into a liquid slurry or a dry powder, formulate the agent with stabilizing chemicals, and fill it into a specialized sprayer device that can disseminate the spores as a fine-particle aerosol, infecting those exposed through the lungs. Outdoor releases of BW agents would also have to timed to take advantage of favorable wind, weather, and atmospheric conditions.

The combination of motivation and technical capabilities required for successful bioterrorism is quite rare. Since 1945, only about a half-dozen terrorist groups have tried to acquire and use biological weapons, and none of them has mastered the complex set of knowledge, skills, and know-how needed to produce and deliver BW agents effectively on a large scale. All known bioterrorist attacks to date have involved standard bacterial or toxin agents (e.g., anthrax spores or ricin) and crude methods of delivery such as the contamination of food, beverages, or unchlorinated water supplies. In 1984, for example, the Rajneeshee cult in Oregon used cultures of salmonella bacteria to taint restaurant salad bars in the town of The Dalles. The attack sickened 751 people, some seriously, but caused no fatalities [3].

In the past, terrorists have faced significant technical problems when attempting to move beyond crude biological weapons, suitable for assassination or food contamination, to more advanced aerosol-delivered agents capable of causing mass casualties. During the early 1990s, for example, the Japanese doomsday cult Aum Shinrikyo prepared a liquid slurry of anthrax spores and dispersed it repeatedly in aerosol form from the roof of a building in Tokyo, but the attacks did not kill or harm anyone. The reason for this failure was that the group had inadvertently acquired, produced, and released a harmless strain of the anthrax bacterium that is used as a veterinary vaccine [8].

Since the U.S.-led invasion of Afghanistan in 2001, Al-Qaeda has become a decentralized global network made up of largely autonomous affiliates in various countries, such as Algeria, Indonesia, and Yemen. These groups appear to lack the expertise and resources needed to organize and carry out a major bioterrorist attack. Although numerous jihadi websites and terrorist manuals provide recipes for producing BW agents such as ricin, they often contain technical errors or yield only crude preparations.

These observations suggest that at least for the near future, the threat of mass-casualty BW attacks will continue to emanate primarily from nation-states. Terrorist attacks with biological weapons, while considerably more likely than state use, will probably remain limited in scale and impact. Nevertheless, a wild card exists that could potentially transform the nature of the BW threat: the potential exploitation of recent advances in the life sciences and biotechnology for hostile purposes.

2.5 Impact of Emerging Biotechnologies

The past few decades have seen a "revolution" in the life sciences that offers great benefits for human health and agriculture but also has potential BW applications. One example is the growing convergence of biological and chemical production technologies [15]. Pharmaceutical companies now use genetically engineered bacteria and yeast to manufacture complex natural products of medicinal interest that are difficult or costly to extract from plant or animal sources. For example, the antimalarial drug artemisinin is currently purified from the sweet wormwood plant. In an attempt to increase the supply of the drug and lower its cost, scientists at the University of California, Berkeley, have used a technique known as "metabolic engineering." They isolated the set of genes coding for enzymes in the biosynthetic pathway of artemisinin from the sweet wormwood plant and inserted them into yeast cells, with the aim of producing an immediate precursor of the drug in large fermentation tanks [11]. In theory, a similar process might be used to mass-produce toxic natural substances such as saxitoxin, a potent paralytic poison made by marine algae that cause harmful blooms known as "red tides." Although at present it is impractical to extract large quantities of saxitoxin from shellfish contaminated by a red tide, metabolic engineering might conceivably be used to mass-produce the toxin for BW purposes.

Also of growing interest to the pharmaceutical industry are bioregulators, natural body chemicals that play a key role in many physiological processes, such as the regulation of temperature, blood pressure, immunity, and brain function. Although these biochemicals are essential for life at extremely low concentrations, they can be toxic at higher doses or when their molecular structure is modified. Neuropeptides, a class of bioregulators in the central nervous system, are known to affect cognition and emotion. These compounds might therefore be developed into a new class of potent incapacitating agents with potential applications in law enforcement, counterinsurgency, and counterterrorist operations. If such biochemical agents prove to be tactically useful, countries might well be motivated to acquire and weaponize them, a development that would seriously undermine the biological and chemical disarmament regimes [14].

Advanced DNA synthesis techniques have also made it possible to reconstitute entire microbial genomes by strictly chemical means, a feat that has been accomplished to date for poliovirus, the 1918 Spanish influenza virus, a SARS-like coronavirus, and a small bacterium [6]. In the future, whole-genome synthesis techniques will make it possible to construct any pathogenic virus for which an accurate genetic sequence has been determined, including the smallpox virus, which was eradicated from nature in the late 1970s by a global vaccination campaign under the auspices of the World Health Organization (WHO). Because smallpox eradication led countries around the world to stop vaccinating their civilian populations against the disease in the early 1980s, the human population has since become increasingly vulnerable to the deliberate use of smallpox as a biological weapon. Although the known stocks of the smallpox virus are currently held at two WHO-approved repositories in the United States and Russia, the CIA reportedly believes that undeclared cashes of the virus may exist in countries of BW proliferation concern, including Russia, Iran, and North Korea [5].

The worldwide diffusion of advanced biotechnologies such as gene synthesis may increase the risk of their misuse for harmful purposes. In principle, terrorists with the necessary scientific training could order fragments of DNA from several commercial suppliers and assemble them into a deadly virus, circumventing the physical access controls on "select agents" of bioterrorism concern. While genome-synthesis technology could be used to recreate known viruses in the laboratory, the design and construction of artificial pathogens more deadly than those that exist in nature will remain unlikely. To create such novel agents, it would be necessary to assemble complexes of genes that work in unison to infect the host and block the human immune response—a task far beyond the current state of the art.

Those individuals who are potentially most capable of harnessing advanced biotechnologies for harmful purposes are life scientists working in academic, industrial, or government labs. Although scientists tend to be highly rational people, the fact that Aum Shinrikyo was able to recruit university-trained biologists and chemists for its unconventional weapons programmes suggests that some brilliant but alienated scientists may be vulnerable to a charismatic leader who provides a false sense of spiritual meaning and community.

The 2001 anthrax letter attacks in the United States have also increased concerns about the so-called "insider" threat. In August 2008, after a 7-year investigation, the Federal Bureau of Investigation (FBI) concluded that the sole perpetrator of the anthrax letter attacks had been Dr. Bruce E. Ivins, a respected microbiologist and developer of anthrax vaccines who had worked for decades at the U.S. Army's premier biodefence laboratory at Fort Detrick in Maryland. Because Ivins committed suicide shortly before he was to be indicted, the evidence against him was never tested in court. Nevertheless, the Ivins case has called attention to the risk that scientists working in national biodefence programmes could be motivated by personal grievance or ideology to carry out biological attacks. Ironically, because the 2001 anthrax letters attacks resulted in a huge expansion of U.S. government biodefence research, today more than 14,000 scientists are authorized to handle "select agents" of bioterrorism concern.

Growing numbers of researchers are also pursuing fields with clear dual-use potential, such as synthetic biology and nanotechnology. The International Genetically Engineered Machines (iGEM) competition, held each year at MIT, attracts student teams from around the world who present research projects involving the manipulation of advanced genetic components and technologies. When the iGEM competition began in 2003, it was limited to a few teams from U.S. universities, but it has since gone global: in 2010, 118 teams from 26 countries participated [17]. Because any large group of people is likely to include some individuals with psychopathic tendencies, the expanding pool of scientists with dual-use knowledge has increased the statistical risk that powerful biotechnologies such as whole-genome synthesis could be misused for harmful purposes.

An important variable in assessing the risk of high-tech bioterrorism is the set of skills and resources needed to acquire and deliver dangerous pathogens effectively. Kathleen Vogel of Cornell University contends that in addition to "explicit knowledge," such as recipes for producing and processing biological agents, would-be bioterrorists would require a great deal of "tacit knowledge" that cannot be written down but must be acquired through hands-on experience in the lab [18]. In addition, the fact that much of the know-how needed to weaponize biological agents remains classified would limit the ability of terrorists lacking specialized training and hands-on experience to prepare mass-casualty attacks.

Other scholars disagree, however, arguing that synthetic genomics and other advanced biotechnologies are subject to a process of "deskilling," or a reduction over time in the level of tacit knowledge required for their use [12]. Genetic engineering techniques that a decade ago could be performed only in cutting-edge laboratories are now available in the form of kits, processes, reagents, and services that can be utilized by individuals with only basic laboratory training. At least potentially, terrorists might also be able to recruit or coerce scientists with prior experience in a state-level BW programme. Given these factors, the risk of high-tech terrorism, while currently low, warrants continued vigilance.

In conclusion, the current bioweapons threat emanates primarily from a few countries of proliferation concern, such as China, Russia, North Korea, and Syria, as well as a small minority of terrorist organizations that are both motivated to acquire and use biological weapons and are technically capable of doing so. At least for the near term, bioterrorist attacks are likely to remain small-scale and to involve standard agents and crude methods of delivery. If, however, terrorist groups manage to move up the technical learning curve, the destructive power of biological attacks could increase significantly.

References

1. Alibek K, Handelman S (1999) Biohazard: the chilling true story of the largest covert biological weapons program in the world—told from inside by the man who ran it. Random House, New York
2. Brogan B (2006) We won't scrap WMD stockpile unless Israel does, says Assad, The Telegraph (London), 6 January 2004
3. Carus WS (2000) The Rajneeshees. In: Tucker JB (ed) Toxic terror: assessing terrorist use of chemical and biological weapons. MIT Press, Cambridge, pp 115–137
4. Drogin B (2007) Curveball: spies, lies, and the con man who caused a war. Random House, New York
5. Gellman B (2002) 4 Nations thought to possess smallpox: Iraq, N. Korea Named, Two Officials Say, Washington Post, 5 November 2002, p A1

6. Gibson DG, Glass JI, Lartigue C et al (2010) Creation of a bacterial cell controlled by a chemically synthesized genome. Science 329:52–56
7. Iraq Survey Group (2004) Comprehensive report of the special advisor to the DCI on Iraq's WMD, 30 September 2004, http://www.gpo.gov/fdsys/pkg/GPO-DUELFERREPORT/content-detail.html. Accessed 20 Sep 2012
8. Kaplan DE (2000) Aum Shinrikyo. In: Tucker JB (ed) Toxic terror: assessing chemical and biological weapons. MIT Press, Cambridge, MA, pp 207–226
9. McCarthy T, Tucker JB (2000) Saddam's toxic arsenal: chemical and biological weapons in the gulf wars. In: Sagan SD, Lavoy PR, Wirtz JJ (eds) Planning the unthinkable. Cornell University Press, Ithaca, pp 47–78
10. Parachini J (2003) Putting WMD terrorism into perspective. Wash Q 26(4):37–50
11. Ro DK, Paradise EM, Ouellet M et al (2006) Production of the antimalarial precursor artemisinic acid in engineered yeast. Nature 440:940–943
12. Schmidt M (2008) Diffusion of synthetic biology: a challenge to biosafety. Syst Synth Biol. doi:10.1007/s11693-008-9018-z
13. Tenet G, Harlow B (2007) At the center of the storm: my years at the CIA. Harper Collins, New York, pp 278–279
14. Tucker JB (2008) The body's own bioweapons. Bull At Sci 64(1):16–22
15. Tucker JB (2010) The convergence of biology and chemistry: implications for arms control verification. Bull At Sci 66(6):56–66
16. U.S. Department of State (2010) Adherence to and compliance with arms control, nonproliferation, and disarmament agreements and commitments. U.S. Department of State, Washington, DC
17. Vinson V (2010) Inventive constructions using biobricks. Science 330(6011):1629
18. Vogel K (2006) Bioweapons proliferation: where science studies and public policy collide. Soc Stud Sci 36(5):659–690

Chapter 3
A New Method of Differentiation Between a Biological Attack and Other Epidemics

Vladan Radosavljevic

Abstract The main obstacle in identifying a biological attack (BA), while preventing false alarms, epidemics of panic and unnecessary expenditures is the insufficient data on which to rely. This new method of outbreak analysis is based on our original model of bioterrorism risk assessment. The intention was to develop a model of quick and accurate evaluation of an unusual epidemiologic event (UEE) that would save time, money, human and material resources and reduce confusion and panic. This UEE analysis is a subtle and detailed differentiation through assessment of BA feasibility in comparison with three other types of outbreak scenarios. There are two types of differences between these four scenarios: qualitative and quantitative. Qualitative and quantitative differences are defined with 23 and 10 indicators, respectively. Both types of indicators can have three different values: N/A, 0 or 1. We have carried out a feasibility analysis for subtle and detailed differentiation among four outbreak scenarios. As a tool for feasibility analysis we have introduced a "system of elimination". System elimination is applied if one component contains all indicators scored with 0 or as N/A – the related scenario is then eliminated from further consideration. The system was applied to four UEEs: (1) an intentional attack by a deliberate use of a biological agent (Amerithrax), (2) a spontaneous outbreak of a new or re-emerging disease ("swine flu"), (3) a spontaneous outbreak by an accidental release of a pathogen (Sverdlovsk anthrax), and (4) a spontaneous natural outbreak of a known endemic disease that may mimic bioterrorism or biowarfare (Kosovo tularemia). It was found that "agent" was the most important and the most informative UEE component of the new scoring system. This system might be helpful in the analysis of unusual epidemic events and a quick differentiation between biological attacks and other epidemics.

V. Radosavljevic (✉)
Military Academy, University of Defence,
Pavla Jurisica Sturma 1, 11000 Belgrade, Serbia

Medical Corps Headquarters, Army of Serbia, Belgrade, Serbia
e-mail: vladanr4@Gmail.Com

I. Hunger et al. (eds.), *Biopreparedness and Public Health: Exploring Synergies*,
NATO Science for Peace and Security Series A: Chemistry and Biology,
DOI 10.1007/978-94-007-5273-3_3,

3.1 Introduction

Most diseases caused by potential biological warfare agents have low natural incidence rates. The lack of clinician experience with these diseases can impede rapid diagnosis and reporting to public health authorities [5]. The main obstacle in identifying a biological attack (BA), while preventing false alarms, epidemics of panic and unnecessary expenditures is the lack of data to rely on [23]. We are trained to consider common causes for syndromes first – and unless we have a high level of suspicion – we may not realize that we need to apply non-standard methods to identify an intentional use and to detect the kind of biological agents that a terrorist might use. Basically, any unexpected occurrence of one or more patients or deaths in humans or animals which might have been caused by an intentional release of pathogens may be the first clue of an unusual epidemic event (UEE). Also, the occurrence of a single case or death caused by an unknown or already eradicated disease or agent may be considered as "unusual".

Three systematic models of assessing differences between natural and deliberate epidemics have been published. Grunow et al. [12] put emphasis on three groups of characteristics: (1) political, military and social analysis of the afflicted region (two criteria), (2) specific features of the pathogen (three criteria), and (3) characteristics of the epidemic and clinical manifestation (six criteria). Dembek et al. [7] proposed 11 potential clues to a deliberate epidemic which are focused on epidemic characteristics. These two models are accurate, but time consuming. However, saving time is crucial in the case of an UEE. Radosavljevic et al. [20]) suggested a model for early orientation and differentiation between natural and deliberate outbreak.

Our new method of outbreak analysis is based on an original model of bioterrorism risk assessment [19]. The intention was to develop a model of quick and accurate evaluation of a UEE that would save time, money, human and material resources and reduce confusion and panic.

This UEE analysis is a subtle and detailed differentiation through assessment of BA feasibility in comparison with other outbreak scenarios, in particular: (1) a spontaneous outbreak of a new or re-emerging disease (NR) (such as "swine flu"), (2) a spontaneous outbreak by an accidental release of a pathogen (AR) (such as the Sverdlovsk anthrax outbreak), and (3) a spontaneous natural outbreak of a known endemic disease that may mimic bioterrorism or biowarfare (NE) (such as the Kosovo tularemia outbreak).

3.2 Subtle and Detailed Differentiation of an UEE

After identification of an UEE we introduced a new method for the subtle and detailed differentiation of such an event. In our previous paper [19] a BA was defined by four components, and now we propose their equivalent terms in an UEE: reservoir/source of infection vs. perpetrator, pathogen vs. biological agent, transmission mechanisms and factors vs. media and means of delivery, and susceptible population vs. target.

Indicators of a deliberate outbreak can be conclusive and non-conclusive [12]. Conclusive indicators are direct and comparatively objective indicators for an intentional event. Non-conclusive indicators estimate only the likelihood of an intentional event on the basis of circumstantial evidence. There are three conclusive indicators of deliberate outbreaks: evidence of intelligence/secrecy activities coincident or related to an outbreak, confirmed presence of a known bio-agent (has characteristics of traditional biological weapons or genetically modified as agent), and evidence of a means of delivery (munitions, delivery systems or dispersion systems). All other indicators are more or less non-conclusive.

3.2.1 Reservoir/Source of Infection vs. Perpetrator

Equivalent to the perpetrator in a biological attack is the source, or reservoir of infection in a natural epidemic. Perpetrators may behave in two ways. Some bioterrorists want to avoid attribution for an attack, others want to claim credit for it, or, at least want the authorities to recognize that a disease outbreak was deliberate, and not of a natural origin. People who are accidentally included in natural outbreaks (as a source or reservoir of infection) and look like perpetrators at first sight, are always highly afraid and cooperative. Also, a source/reservoir of infection always completely behaves according to epidemiological characteristics (incubation period, period of communicability) [18].

If political, military, ethnic, religious or other motives can be identified, this would lend credence to the assumption that an attack using pathogens or toxins as biological agents has taken place. In natural outbreaks usually there is no motive, but if we find them, motive(s) are commonplace and simple. In natural epidemics sources of infection may be discovered by usual epidemiological and microbiological routine investigations, and there are no tendencies to keep themselves unknown (no secrecy) [19].

There are some coincident points related to an outbreak that may be an indicator of secrecy/intelligence inclusion in a biological attack. Intelligence presents an ability to get true and on-time information on a global and local level related to biological attacks [19]. If some activities related to a biological attack are kept unobserved before an attack as well as after an attack, it is a parameter of secrecy and should be considered in the context of a biological attack. It would also be conceivable that certain persons or groups may be given sufficient prior warning about a biological attack and could have been spared from an epidemic by preventive measures (e.g. receiving vaccinations, adhering strictly to instructions to boil drinking water).

Quantitative parameters. In natural outbreaks the number and distribution of sources of infection are related to the incubation period and period of disease communicability. Such regularity is seldom seen in a biological attack. Here we also have to consider special situations in natural outbreaks when the incubation times and communicability may be changed: for instance in the case of an exposure to massive doses of pathogens by contaminated water or food, such as may be the case with natural disasters or accidents in water treatment plants and distribution systems or hygienic failures in kitchens. Then we may have epidemiological, microbiological and clinical patterns which could resemble the characteristics we would also expect in a biological attack.

Strategic (large-scale) biological attack. States' institutions such as military forces, intelligence services or well-funded and possibly state-supported organizations can be perpetrators in a strategic biological attack. The present threat analysis states that in the next years only a very few so called "rogue" countries with clandestine offensive biological warfare programmes would be able to launch strategic biological attacks [19]. Such attacks include politically, military and/or ideologically motivated ones. In natural, large-scale epidemics, infection is mainly unintentionally and individually disseminated and strictly related through periods of incubation and communicability of disease. The period between deployment of a bioweapon and its effects, however, is long enough to give a terrorist a chance to escape. So, it could be very difficult to find a perpetrator.

Operational (middle-scale) biological attack. This type of attack could be carried out by all three types of perpetrators (government supported institutions/organizations, terrorist groups, individuals) [19]. If psychological effects (fear and panic) are greater than the biological losses (diseased and died) it might also be a biological attack [21, 22].

Tactical (small-scale) biological attack. The terrorist or criminal groups dominate as perpetrators in this type of attack. If "hard" targets are hit, perpetrators likely have to be highly skilled, or with suicidal tendencies, and politically or ideologically motivated [19].

Qualitative indicators. Qualitative indicators related to BA have no equivalents (not applicable – N/A) in two cases: natural outbreak of a known endemic disease that may mimic bioterrorism (biowarfare), or outbreak of a new or re-emerging disease. In the case of an accidental release of a pathogen, motivation, ability and intelligence information are N/A.

Three quantitative indicators of a BA have their equivalents in the other three outbreak scenarios – AR, NE and NR.

3.2.2 Pathogen vs. Biological Agent

The most difficult scenario of a BA for investigators is if an endemic pathogen was used. In such a case microbial forensic tools for identifying a deliberate outbreak should be given priority.

Type of agent. There are two types of biological agents: conventional (natural form of the pathogen) and biological warfare agent. A qualitative parameter may be if some pathogen species or strain (subspecies) is unusual, atypical or antiquated, e.g. is identified in the region concerned for the first time ever or again after a long absence, or if an agent has certain characteristics like: a special genetic signature, mixed with a stabilizing agent, highly concentrated, filled in munitions, high toxicity, more virulent, resistant to antibiotics, and multiple modes of transmission. Many potential biological warfare agents could be obtained from natural sources (infected animals, patients, or contaminated soil). Many pathogens, perhaps the majority concerned, cause zoonoses, i.e. infect animals as well as humans [16]. The sudden occurrence of a zoonotic disease, such as brucellosis, in the absence of the natural animal host or reservoir and other likely sources of transmission may be suggestive of an unnatural cause. The so-called "zoonotic" potential should be considered in this differentiating evaluation. A regionalized animal die-off may provide a clue that something is present or may have been released that might also infect humans. This phenomenon of animal illness heralding human illness was observed during the West Nile virus encephalitis outbreak in New York City in 1999, when many local crows, along with exotic birds at the Bronx Zoo, died [17, 24]. In the case of a so-called "reverse spread", where human disease precedes animal disease, or human and animal disease occur simultaneously, one should consider an unnatural spread. This is often also the case in plague or tularemia outbreaks and has led to speculations like in Surat (India) in 1994 or Kosovo. Many strains isolated from nature have low virulence. Therefore, a terrorist must isolate many different strains before finding one sufficiently potent as a warfare agent. Considering the technical difficulties to obtain virulent microorganisms from nature, terrorists may find it easier to steal well-characterized strains from a research laboratory, or to purchase the known pathogenic strains from a national culture collection or commercial supplier. Between 1985 and 1989, the Iraqi government ordered virulent strains of anthrax and other pathogens from culture collections in France and the United States, presumably for public health research – a purpose that was legal at the time, and approved by the U.S. Department of Commerce [25, 26]. It is speculated that one reason for the lack of success in causing illness following dissemination of anthrax spores by the cult Aum Shinrikyo was the inadvertent selection of a non-pathogenic strain of *Bacillus anthracis* [14].

Strategic (large-scale) biological attack. Respiratory agents are almost always candidates for strategic use because of the possibility for their clandestine use, their high dispersal potential, and their high contagiousness. Category A agents, and the agents causing SARS, avian influenza, and pandemic influenza (including swine flu) might be candidates for use at the strategic level [19].

Operational (middle-scale) biological attack. For this type of attack, the spectrum of suitable agents is wider than for large-scale attacks, and possibilities include (in addition to the agents mentioned above) Hanta viruses, multi drug resistant *Mycobacterium tuberculosis*, hepatitis A virus, Noroviruses, *Cryptosporidium spp.*, and toxins [19]. Consequently, measures of detection and identification are more difficult. Also, the accessibility of these agents for terrorists is easier, and the amounts of the available agent are larger.

Tactical (small-scale) biological attack. The agents from all three categories and emerging biological agents are potential candidates for this purpose. Biological agents are still the preferred materials of hoax perpetrators at the tactical level, probably because perpetrators could easily produce and safely handle these simulants of potential biological warfare agents.

Amount of agent. If there is a non-proportional, large amount of biological agent present in sources/reservoirs or environmental sampling, or an epidemiologically unexplainable transmission or distribution of an agent, there is a high probability of a biological attack.

All four outbreak scenarios could have the same values for indicators related to agent.

3.2.3 Transmission Mechanisms and Factors vs. Media and Means of Delivery

If we find some kind of munition, delivery system or dispersion system (means of delivery) at the outbreak focus it should be the proof of a deliberate epidemic. If food, water, or fomites are the media of delivery it should be possible to trace it and find out the source of infection and type (natural or artificial) of epidemic. But, air as a medium of delivery remains the most complicated for investigation. Looking for people who came in contact with the agent through this method of exposure may be very difficult. However, several other parameters may help (type, strain and approximate amount of released agent, period of incubation, and period of communicability). Also, natural epidemics will feature paths of transmission that are typical for the pathogen and its natural hosts. Such deviations from natural paths of infection could indicate that biological agents have been deliberately disseminated. Many diseases exhibit vastly different clinical presentations, periods of incubation, and mortality rates depending upon the route of transmission. Therefore, outbreaks due to an atypical route of transmission, particularly aerosol transmission, such as in the inhalation anthrax example above, are more suggestive of an intentional use. Weather factors, especially wind direction, temperature, and humidity, are important determinants of pathogen dissemination and disease occurrence and must be taken into account in an outbreak investigation. A disease outbreak occurring downwind (or downriver) of a suspected biological warfare agent production facility, such as in the Sverdlovsk anthrax disaster, provides compelling evidence for an accidental or intentional release [27]. It is useful to plot locations where cases occur on a geographic map. If affected cases are clustered in a downwind pattern, an aerosol release should be considered like in the 1979 anthrax outbreak in Sverdlovsk [7].

Many people are becoming increasingly mobile and interactive with indigenous populations. As a result, they have a correspondingly greater potential for translocating diseases to previously non-endemic areas through unknown transportation of infected vectors or people during incubation or clinical symptom stages. Therefore, knowledge of the at-risk population's travel and contact histories may be essential in determining the etiology and likely source of an outbreak. Tourists, military personnel, traders, settlers and immigrants, and travel adventurers may carry new pathogens to unsuspecting and susceptible populations. People, storms, and floods can transport arthropods, rodents, snails, birds, and other creatures that can also bring new infections to previously unaffected areas. Changes in human behaviour, technologic devices, the environment, institutional living, and poor nutrition or vitamin deficits can spark new epidemics. The speed at which an epidemic spreads is determined by the virulence, resistance and concentration of the pathogen, the contagiousness of the disease and the intensity of the transmission process, on the one hand, and on the susceptibility and disposition of the exposed population, on the other. It is unclear how changes in household sizes, working patterns, and mobility would affect transmission patterns today. Incorporating detailed data on demographics and human mobility into spatially explicit models offers one method by which such extrapolation can be made more reliable, but the scale of changes mean that much uncertainty will inevitably remain.

Qualitative indicators: Air, water, food and fomites could be the media or means of delivery for all four outbreak scenarios.

Quantitative indicators: Three quantitative indicators of BA – munitions, delivery systems, and dispersion systems – will not exist in the other three UEE scenarios – AR, NE, and NR.

3.2.4 Susceptible Population vs. Target

In natural outbreaks there is no target, but there is a susceptible (affected or endangered) population. In both natural and deliberate epidemics there can be two types of consequences: direct (death and/or illness), and indirect (political and economic). However, in a deliberate outbreak, indirect (political and economic) effects are usually intended and have great impact. In natural epidemics indirect (political and economic) effects every time are "collateral damage" or sometimes expected consequences of disasters. In addition, the use and even the threatened use of certain biological agents can have intense psychological effects on the population at large [19, 21].

In naturally occurring epidemics "soft" targets are mainly affected, because "hard" targets (e.g. heads of state or other VIPs) are better protected than "soft" targets (e.g. the unprotected population). There are no signs or indicators of intelligence/secret activities (e.g. repeated visits by individuals or vehicles identified as out of place, prior warning of a possible biological attack such as active or passive immunoprophylaxis or chemo-prophylaxis of a non-target population, threats, or hoaxes). There is no suspicious behaviour: unexplained contamination of a media (air, food, and water), or use of unusual fomites (office equipment, postal letters). There is also no obvious target in a natural outbreak. Some parameters of an outbreak (location of the exposure/target site, importance and number of people in the site, and distribution of people from the site) may also point to a deliberate attack.

Large-scale attack. Nowadays, one of the main objectives of a bioterrorist is to propagate fear, anxiety, uncertainty, and depression within the population, induce mistrust of the government, inflict economic damage, and disrupt travel and commerce [19, 21]. Causing significant outbreaks of disease may be a secondary objective. The ultimate goal of biological attacks is to cause political consequences. Bioterrorists want to produce an epidemic of fear and panic [19, 21]. This cannot be evoked in such manner if the attack is clandestine and mimics a natural outbreak. Naturally occurring large-scale epidemics or pandemics are only possible by aerosol transmissible agents. All other large-scale outbreaks should raise suspicion as a potential deliberate outbreak.

Middle-scale and small-scale attack. In the case of "hard targets" (highly prominent and protected institutions like governmental buildings, media centres, and persons such as politicians, scientist, or high military officials) being affected, the probability of a deliberate outbreak is high. Consequences even in small-scale attacks can be of strategic importance. "Soft targets" are considered ordinary people in public places (e.g. respiratory agents in crowded and closed places like theatres, cinemas, sports events, and political meetings). Small-scale outbreaks in "soft targets" are more difficult to differentiate and may be of less strategic importance.

Except for the most blatant violations of natural principles, bioterrorism will continue to remain difficult to differentiate from naturally occurring outbreaks. Certain attributes of a disease outbreak, while perhaps not pathognomonic for a biological attack when considered singly, may in combination with other attributes provide convincing evidence for intentional causation. The possibility of mixed epidemics must always be taken into consideration when assessing the outbreak of a disease, since they complicate the epidemiologic situation and can present additional difficulties for the investigation of unusual outbreaks.

3.2.5 General Differentiating and Scoring

There are two types of differences between these four scenarios: qualitative and quantitative. Qualitative differences are defined by 23 indicators, and quantitative by ten indicators. Both types of indicators could have three different values: N/A, 0, or 1.

In our previous article [19] numerous parameters – indicators were defined. By using them we have carried out feasibility analysis for subtle and detailed differentiation among four outbreak scenarios. As a tool for feasibility analysis we have introduced a "system of elimination". System elimination is necessitated if one component contains all indicators scored with 0 or as N/A, then the related scenario is eliminated from further consideration.

3.3 Examples of Different Outbreak Scenarios (Table 3.1)

3.3.1 Spontaneous Outbreak of a New or Re-Emerging Disease (Swine Flu)

Reservoirs. Reservoirs of infection are pigs [4, 6, 9] and turkeys, and all six qualitative indicators are not applicable (NE, NR scenarios). In consideration of BA scenario there are likely no terrorists who intend to create an uncontrolled pandemic originating in a Mexico rural area. Later events also showed that there was no misuse or intent either for commercial purposes by pharmaceutical industries or from military experiments. Therefore this scenario has been eliminated. With pigs and turkeys as the reservoir, accidental release of the pathogen is also not likely, and therefore this scenario is eliminated.

Agent. Undoubtedly, this is a new and emerging pathogen [6, 10]. This clearly eliminates a natural outbreak of a known endemic disease.

Transmission mechanisms and devices vs. media and means of delivery. Air and fomites could be the media of delivery in a new or a re-emerging disease [1, 2, 13, 15].

Susceptible population vs. target. In the "swine flu" pandemic, intelligence and secrecy are both scored with 1 because of the early detection of the outbreak, and identification of the agent and reservoirs of infection.

Conclusion. "System elimination" clearly discriminates a spontaneous natural outbreak of a known endemic disease, a biological attack, outbreak by an accidental release of a pathogen because they do not have the components "agent" or "perpetrator". Considering the first component (perpetrator or reservoirs/sources) in the third scenario, the first six qualitative indicators are N/A. The three quantitative indicators are each scored 1. Taking into account the scores of 1 for intelligence and secrecy, as well as the absolute absence of material evidence of biological attack, we should accept the scenario as a spontaneous outbreak of a new or re-emerging disease.

Emerging diseases, both new to a region like West Nile virus encephalitis, and totally "new" like SARS and avian influenza, have occurred in the last decade. Examples include the appearance of West Nile virus encephalitis in New York City in 1999 [8], bubonic plague cases in New York City in 2002 [3], or monkey pox outbreak in the USA in 2003.

The West Nile virus encephalitis outbreak in New York City in 1999 constituted a true emerging infection, as the disease became established in a new location, while the plague cases were simply imported by out-of-state residents. Until the epidemic in New York City in 1999, West Nile virus had never been isolated in the Western hemisphere. Many diseases, such as dengue fever in Cuba having been imported from Vietnam, or vivax malaria in Korea, represent a re-establishment of endemic transmission in areas from which they were once eradicated. About 40 new pathogens have been found in the last 35 years [11]. The United States was caught off-guard by the

Table. 3.1 Assessment of four unusual epidemiologic events by a differentiation scoring

	Swine flu				Amerithrax				Kosovo tularemia				Sverdlovsk anthrax			
Parameter	BA	NE	NR	AR	BA	NE	NR	AR	BA	NE	NR	AR	BA	NE	NR	AR
Perpetrator																
Source/Reservoir of infection																
Sophistication	0	N/A	N/A	0	1	N/A	N/A	0	0	N/A	N/A	0	1	0	0	1
Motivation/Intention	0	N/A	N/A	0	1	N/A	N/A	0	1	N/A	N/A	0	1	0	0	0
Ability	0	N/A	N/A	0	1	N/A	N/A	0	0	N/A	N/A	0	0	0	0	1
Capacity	0	N/A	N/A	0	1	N/A	N/A	0	0	N/A	N/A	0	0	0	0	1
Intelligence	0	N/A	N/A	0	1	N/A	N/A	0	0	N/A	N/A	0	1	0	0	1
Secrecy	0	N/A	N/A	0	1	N/A	N/A	0	0	N/A	N/A	0	0	0	0	1
Number of perpetrators / sources / reservoirs	0	1	1	0	1	0	0	0	0	1	1	0	1	0	0	1
Accessibility to sources of agent	0	1	1	0	1	0	0	0	0	1	1	0	1	0	0	1
Accessibility to targets	0	1	1	0	1	0	0	0	0	0	1	0	1	0	0	1
Agent																
Pathogen																
A category	–	0	0	–	1	–	–	–	1	1	0	–	1	–	–	1
B category	–	0	0	–	0	–	–	–	0	0	0	–	0	–	–	0
C category	–	0	0	–	0	–	–	–	0	0	0	–	0	–	–	0
Emerging agent	–	0	1	–	0	–	–	–	0	0	0	–	0	–	–	0
Amount of the available agent	–	0	1	–	1	–	–	–	1	1	0	–	1	–	–	1
Means/Media of delivery																
Transmission mechanisms																
Air	–	–	1	–	1	–	–	–	0	1	–	–	1	–	–	1
Food	–	–	0	–	0	–	–	–	0	1	–	–	0	–	–	0
Water	–	–	0	–	0	–	–	–	0	1	–	–	0	–	–	0
Fomites	–	–	1	–	1	–	–	–	0	1	–	–	0	–	–	0

Vectors	–	–	0	–	0	–	–	–	0	1	–	–	0	–	–	0
Munition	–	–	0	–	0	–	–	–	0	0	–	–	0	–	–	0
Delivery systems	–	–	0	–	1	–	–	–	0	0	–	–	0	–	–	0
Dispersion systems	–	–	0	–	0	–	–	–	0	0	–	–	0	–	–	0
Target																
Susceptible population																
Intelligence	–	–	1	–	1	–	–	–	0	1	–	–	0	–	–	1
Secrecy	–	–	1	–	1	–	–	–	0	0	–	–	1	–	–	1
Personal control	–	–	0	–	1	–	–	–	0	0	–	–	1	–	–	1
Control of means / media	–	–	0	–	1	–	–	–	0	0	–	–	1	–	–	1
Physical protection	–	–	0	–	1	–	–	–	0	0	–	–	1	–	–	1
Protection by chemo-prophylaxis	–	–	0	–	1	–	–	–	0	0	–	–	1	–	–	1
Protection by immuno-prophylaxis	–	–	0	–	1	–	–	–	0	0	–	–	1	–	–	1
Importance of target	–	–	1	–	1	–	–	–	0	1	–	–	0	–	–	1
Number of people in a target	–	–	1	–	1	–	–	–	0	1	–	–	0	–	–	1
Distribution of people in a target	–	–	1	–	1	–	–	–	0	1	–	–	0	–	–	1
Location of target	–	–	1	–	1	–	–	–	0	1	–	–	0	–	–	1
Total	0	3	**13**	0	**25**	0	0	0	3	**15**	3	0	15	0	0	**22**

BA Biological attack, *NE* Natural epidemic, *NR* Outbreak of a new or re-emerging disease, *AR* Accidental release of a pathogen
0 = Low probability, 1 = High probability, N/A = not applicable, – = Eliminated from further consideration
Total: 0–8 = Lowly probable type of outbreak, 9–16 = Possible type of outbreak, 17–24 = Highly probable type of outbreak, 25–33 = Certain type of outbreak

increasing AIDS epidemic that began in the early 1980s. Today, the AIDS epidemic – at the beginning of the twenty-first century – is worse than the worst-case scenarios that were predicted in the early 1990s. Tuberculosis, re-emerged in the United States in the 1980s after decades of decline, and includes newer multidrug-resistant strains.

3.3.2 Intentional Attack by Deliberate Use of a Biological Agent (Amerithrax)

Perpetrator. There were repeated and separate BAs using this agent (e.g. multiple letters sent), which is not very probable in an accidental release.

Agent. The causative agent in this scenario is a category A agent (Ames strain from the US Army Medical Research Institute for Infectious Diseases, Fort Detrick) that was misused by an experienced insider and specially prepared and released deliberately in a significant amount. Because of this, a natural outbreak of a known endemic disease and a spontaneous outbreak of a new or re-emerging disease are clearly eliminated from further consideration.

Transmission mechanisms and devices vs. media and means of delivery. The perpetrator used postal letters (fomites) and the American Postal Service (delivery system) for the BA.

Susceptible population vs. target. Three indicators – intelligence, secrecy and personal control (of employees with access to the agent) – were not successfully applied at the initial phase of the BA. Intelligence is a cornerstone of prevention. Information is provided using electronic surveillance methods, local intelligence systems, and observation of possible targets. Repeated visits by individuals or vehicles must be identified. The impact of secrecy has been evident in some recent incidents. Such an incident occurred in the aftermath of the 2001 anthrax letter attacks. Although the US Postal Service and the CDC knew that the Brentwood postal facility in Washington, D.C., was contaminated, they waited for 4 days before closing the facility and treating workers with antibiotics. By that time, one worker had died of anthrax, another was close to death, and two were gravely ill. Another example is China in 2003, when the government denied the SARS epidemic for 6 weeks, causing international alarm and spread of the disease. These examples illustrate that government secrecy is a persistent jeopardy, leaves the public in ignorance, and allows narrow-minded political agendas to undermine healthcare goals. Personal control includes physical control of people (their health status) and behavioral control (CV review, control of suspect behavior, control of contacts) [19].

Conclusion. "System elimination" clearly eliminates the other three scenarios by the "agent" and "perpetrator" components. Therefore, we should accept the BA scenario as the likely event.

During 1900–2001, 77 biological "events" (i.e. episodes involving the deliberate use of a biological agent to harm people) were perpetrated. Of these, just four post-1945 events generated more than ten casualties [28]. Besides this, about a thousand anthrax hoaxes occurred alone between 1996 and 2001 which concerned the public, administration, and public health authorities, prompting excessive decontamination and post-exposure measures and intensive forensic and laboratory investigations in order to discriminate the events as false alarms.

3.3.3 Spontaneous Natural Outbreak of a Known Endemic Disease That May Mimic Bioterrorism or Biowarfare (Kosovo Tularemia Outbreak)

Reservoirs/sources. In the Kosovo tularemia outbreak, only an insider could be a possible perpetrator as others would not have the ability or knowledge because of the unpredictable war and after-war events. The secrecy and capacity needed would be possible only from highly sophisticated insiders. The qualitative indicators from BA and natural epidemic scenarios are not similar (rodents were reservoirs) and their differences are assessed in the rest of the indicators. Quantitative indicators are also different. The number of perpetrators should be numerous but were not identified, however the number of rodents as reservoirs were numerous. Comparing the accessibility to sources of the agent with the distribution sources of the agent, as well as accessibility to the target by perpetrators (humans) and rodents as reservoirs, there are significant differences. Because of the timing and geographically very dispersed occurrence of cases, quantitative indicators related to a perpetrator were scored with 0, and those related to a natural epidemic were scored with 1. A spontaneous outbreak by an accidental release of a pathogen and BA were not likely scenarios because of the timing, geographic separation, and repeated occurrence of cases.

Agent. The implicated agent was *Francisella tularensis holarctica*, that causes a milder form of tularemia and is endemic in the Balkan region. Because of this, a spontaneous outbreak of a new or re-emerging disease is clearly eliminated.

Transmission mechanisms and devices vs. media and means of delivery. There was no convincing and conclusive evidence for devices of delivery [12]. It is well known tularemia could be spread by multiple natural transmission sources like water, food, or animals, as was the case in this outbreak.

Susceptible population vs. target. This component should provide the final information to solve the conundrum between a BA and a natural epidemic scenario. There was no intelligence information (no convincing or conclusive indicator was documented regarding a possible perpetrator), no secrecy (no attempts to control information after the first diagnosed cases), no control of means/media, no physical protection, chemical protection, or immunological protection (all three types of protection and ways to control transmission were absent or implemented late), and a lack of significance from a military/terrorist BA logistical standpoint in the importance and location of the target, and the number and distribution of the people affected.

Conclusion. "System elimination" clearly excluded a spontaneous outbreak of a new or re-emerging disease because of the agent type (not new or re-emerging). The scenario of spontaneous outbreak by an accidental release of a pathogen was also not likely because of timing, geographic dispersion, and repeated occurrence of cases without any convincing and conclusive indicator. The total score supports a scenario of a spontaneous natural outbreak of a known endemic disease that could mimic bioterrorism or bio-warfare.

3.3.4 Spontaneous Outbreak by an Accidental Release of a Pathogen (Sverdlovsk Anthrax Outbreak)

Perpetrator. In the Sverdlovsk anthrax outbreak, the large amount of agent (enough to contaminate a city with thousands of inhabitants and the surrounding area) was not likely spread from a natural source or reservoir of infection unobserved and in such a short time. These facts eliminate two scenarios: natural epidemic and a spontaneous outbreak of a new or re-emerging disease. Regarding the circumstances in the 1960s in the former Soviet Union with an isolated city (Sverdlovsk) in Siberia, for a BA scenario, capacity and secrecy are scored with 0.

Agent. There was a large amount of spores of a virulent strain of *Bacillus anthracis* (Category A agent) as the causative agent. Accordingly, we scored those two indicators with 1.

Transmission mechanisms and devices vs. media and means of delivery. There were no delivery devices identified. However, the only way to spread such large quantities of anthrax spores during this short period of time was by air.

Susceptible population vs. target. This component should solve the doubt between a BA and accidental pathogen release scenario. In terms of intelligence, no conclusive or inconclusive perpetrator activities or other evidence related to BA were documented, but there was very conclusive evidence related to an accidental release. In terms of secrecy, there was prolonged and stringent secrecy and disinformation supported by Soviet officials about the event. Personal control, control of means/media, physical protection, chemical protection, immunological protection were carried out quickly. The last four indicators – importance of target, number of people in the target, distribution of people in the target, and location of target – were without significance and any military/terrorist logic in a BA scenario. An accidental release scenario was possible, especially accounting for the circumstances (military compound dealing with production of a biological warfare agent close to the city).

Conclusion. "System elimination" clearly eliminates a natural epidemic and a spontaneous outbreak of a new or re-emerging disease through the perpetrator/sources/reservoirs component. Large amounts of the agent in the Sverdlovsk anthrax outbreak were not possible from natural sources/reservoirs of infection in such a short time and would not likely have been otherwise undetected before human cases occurred.

The total score supports a scenario of a spontaneous outbreak by an accidental release of a pathogen as the most likely scenario. Also, if a country rejects foreign help and experts and hides the circumstances of an epidemic it could raise suspicion for an accidental release epidemic scenario.

3.4 General Conclusion

The author has developed a new scoring method of outbreak analysis: for subtle and detailed differentiation. The method was applied to four UEEs: (1) an intentional attack by a deliberate use of a biological agent (Amerithrax), (2) a spontaneous outbreak of a new or re-emerging disease ("swine flu"), (3) a spontaneous outbreak by an accidental release of a pathogen (Sverdlovsk anthrax), and (4) a spontaneous natural outbreak of a known endemic disease that may mimic bioterrorism or biowarfare (Kosovo tularemia). It was found that "agent" was the most important and the most informative UEE component of the new scoring method. This method might be helpful in the analysis of unusual epidemic events and a quick way to differentiate between biological attacks and other epidemics.

References

1. Bean B, Moore B, Sterner B, Petersen L, Gerding DN, Balfour HH Jr (1982) Survival of influenza viruses on environmental surfaces. J Infect Dis 146:47–51
2. Boone SA, Gerba CP (2005) The occurrence of influenza A virus on house hold and day care center fomites. J Infect 51:103–109
3. Centers for Disease Control and Prevention (2002) Imported plague – New York City, 2002. Morb Mort Wkly Rep 52:725–728
4. Centers for Disease Control and Prevention (2009) Serum cross-reactive antibody response to a novel influenza A (H1N1) virus after vaccination with seasonal influenza vaccine. Morb Mortal Wkly Rep 58:521–524
5. Chang M, Glynn MK, Groseclose SL (2003) Endemic, notifiable bioterrorism-related diseases, United States, 1992–1999. Emerg Infect Dis 9:556–564
6. Dawood FS, Jain S, Finelli L et al (2009) Emergence of a novel swine-origin influenza A (H1N1) virus in humans. N Engl J Med 360:2605–2615
7. Dembek ZF, Kortepeter MG, Pavlin JA (2007) Discernment between deliberate and natural infectious disease outbreaks. Epidemiol Infect 135:353–371
8. Fin A, Layton M (2001) Lessons from the West Nile viral encephalitis outbreak in New York City, 1999: implications for bioterrorism preparedness. Clin Infect Dis 32:277–282
9. Fraser C, Donnelly CA, Cauchemez S et al (2009) Pandemic potential of a strain of influenza A (H1N1): early findings. Science 324:1557–1561
10. Gatherer D (2009) The 2009 H1N1 influenza outbreak in its historical context. J Clin Virol 45:174–178
11. Greenberg MI, Marty AM (2006) Emerging natural threats and the deliberate use of biological agents. Clin Lab Med 26:287–298
12. Grunow R, Finke EJ (2002) A procedure for differentiating between the intentional release of biological warfare agents and natural outbreaks of disease: its use in analyzing the tularemia outbreak in Kosovo in 1999 and 2000. Clin Microbiol Infect 8:510–521

13. Gutiırrez I, Litzroth A, Hammadi S et al (2009) Community transmission of influenza A (H1N1) virus at a rock festival in Belgium, 2–5 July 2009. Euro Surveill 14:19294
14. Haas CN (2002) The role of risk analysis in understanding bioterrorism. Risk Anal 22:671–677
15. Hayden F, Coriser A (2005) Transmission of avian influenza viruses to and between humans. J Infect Dis 192:1311–1314
16. Last JM (1988) A dictionary of epidemiology. Oxford University Press, New York
17. Ludwig GW, Calle PP, Mangiafico JA, Raphael BL, Danner DK, Hile JA (2002) An outbreak of West Nile virus in a New York City captive wildlife population. Am J Trop Med Hyg 67:67–75
18. Radosavljevic V (2011) Environmental health and bioterrorism. In: Nriagu JO (ed) Encyclopedia of environmental health, vol 2. Elsevier, Burlington, pp 392–399
19. Radosavljevic V, Belojevic G (2009) A new model of bioterrorism risk assessment. Biosecur Bioterror 7:443–451
20. Radosavljevic V, Belojevic G (2012) Unusual epidemiological event – new model for early orientation and differentation between natural and deliberate outbreak. Public Health 126:77–81
21. Radosavljevic V, Jakovljevic B (2007) Bioterrorism – types of epidemics, new epidemiological paradigm and levels of prevention. Public Health 121:549–557
22. Radosavljevic V, Radunovic D, Belojevic G (2009) Epidemics of panic during a bioterrorist attack – a mathematical model. Med Hypotheses 73:342–346
23. Schultz CH (2004) Chinese curses, anthrax, and the risk of bioterrorism. Ann Emerg Med 43:329–332
24. Steele KE, Linn MJ, Schoepp RJ, Komar N, Geisbert TW, Manduca RM (2000) Pathology of fatal West Nile virus infections in native and exotic birds during the 1999 outbreak in New York City, New York. Vet Pathol 37:208–224
25. Tucker JB (2003) Biosecurity: limiting terrorist access to deadly pathogens. Peaceworks No. 52, United States Institute of Peace. www.usip.org/files/resources/pwks52.pdf. Accessed 19 Feb 2012
26. US Senate Committee on Banking, Housing and Urban Affairs (1994) United States dual-use exports to Iraq and their impact on the health of the Persian Gulf War Veterans. 103rd Congress 2nd session, : U.S. Government Printing Office, Washington DC, pp 266–275
27. Woods CW, Ospanov K, Myrzabekov A, Favorov M, Plikaytis B, Ashford DA (2004) Risk factors for human anthrax among contacts of anthrax-infected livestock in Kazakhstan. Am J Trop Med Hyg 71:48–52
28. Zilinskas RA, Hope B, North DW (2004) A discussion of findings and their possible implications from a workshop on bioterrorism threat assessment and risk management. Risk Anal 24:901–908

Chapter 4
The Difference in Responding to Natural and Unnatural Outbreaks

Amesh A. Adalja

Abstract The response to natural and unnatural outbreaks share many elements. However, unnatural outbreak management will consist of several additional tasks: nuanced communication strategies, concomitant forensic investigations, consideration of altered pathogen features, and bioremediation concerns.

4.1 Introduction

The response to any outbreak – natural or unnatural – will have many response elements that are identical because what is being responded to, in either case, is an infectious disease. The strengths in responding to one type of an outbreak will impact the strength in responding to the other. However, important differences in responding to an unnatural outbreak exist and include: anticipating the virulence of the organism, consideration of engineered pathogen strains, coordinating a concomitant forensic investigation, communication strategies, and planning for bioremediation.

4.2 An Unnatural Outbreak Masquerading as a Natural Outbreak

To concretize what an unnatural outbreak consists of and to emphasize how response plans are, in many ways, identical exploring the case of the intentional *Salmonella* contamination of restaurants in Wasco County, Oregon (USA) in 1984 is instructive.

A.A. Adalja (✉)
Center for Biosecurity, University of Pittsburgh
Medical Center, Baltimore, MD, USA
e-mail: aadalja@upmc-biosecurity.org

I. Hunger et al. (eds.), *Biopreparedness and Public Health: Exploring Synergies*,
NATO Science for Peace and Security Series A: Chemistry and Biology,
DOI 10.1007/978-94-007-5273-3_4,

In September of 1984 in Wasco County, patrons of a local pizza restaurant developed the signs and symptoms of gastroenteritis which on 17 September were reported to the local health department. Within a few days, over 20 cases had been discovered and one patient's stool culture had revealed *Salmonella*. The *Salmonella* strain isolated was sensitive to all antimicrobials, an uncommon feature in strains from the area. In fact, during the past 3 years' 16 prior cases this strain did not appear. The appearance of a novel strain causing many cases signified that a new outbreak of *Salmonella* with a geographically novel strain was underway.

A second wave of illness 1 week later sickened 586 restaurant patrons from ten different restaurants. At this point, the US Centers for Disease Control and Prevention (CDC) was invited by local authorities to investigate the outbreak. Analysis of the outbreak victims revealed a common link: eating from a salad bar. Consequently, salad bar service was halted. As some food handlers were also sick, investigation of food handling practices ensued without any clear evidence of lapses in hygiene. Moreover, salad bar temperatures, dairy sources, water sources, and farms did not reveal any aberrancy and there was no common source for the food on the salad bar. *Salmonella* was found in salad dressing but not in the ingredients, indicating contamination after preparation. Similarly, *Salmonella* was found in coffee creamer milk, but not the constituent milk. The "official" report attributed the 1,000 person outbreak to lapses in food handling practices.

Approximately 1 year later – after a member of a religious cult had a disagreement with another member – it was revealed that the *Salmonella* outbreak had been an intentional act orchestrated by the Rajneeshee cult as a trial run of a plan to influence voter turnout at an upcoming election. The *Salmonella* had been obtained from a commercial supplier and laboratories operated by the cult were used to prepare the bacteria for dissemination.

This intentional attack was managed entirely as if it were unintentional, and it was only in retrospect that it was confirmed to be an act of bioterrorism. Early suspicions of bioterrorism were considered and dismissed because no motive was apparent, no claims of responsibility were offered, no unusual behavior patterns at restaurants were apparent, and no disgruntled employees were identified [7].

4.3 Unnatural Outbreaks 101

As the *Salmonella* case illustrates, many similarities in the response to an intentional outbreak, albeit one that was not recognized as such, exist. The strengths, and more importantly the weaknesses, of a response to a natural outbreak will directly impact the ability to respond to intentional outbreaks. Preparation by physicians, public health entities, and governments for natural outbreaks will also serve as partial preparation for an intentional outbreak as the initial steps in both cases will be identical.

Ascertaining that an outbreak has occurred, developing a case definition, enumerating cases, developing a countermeasure (vaccines and antimicrobials) strategy, and public health messaging will all be very similar in either type of outbreaks. It is only after certain "red flags" are noticed, likely after initial diagnostic steps have been taken, that the response may change.

Certain clues that may signal an unnatural outbreak include the severity of disease, the scale of the outbreak, the time course of the outbreak, and the pathogen identified [4]. However, these clues are not iron-clad nor a guarantee of labeling an outbreak correctly, as the sentinel case of the 2001 anthrax attacks in the US was initially labeled as a natural [6].

Once an outbreak has been identified or suspected to be unnatural or intentional, several actions will be called for by policy makers and the public. Paramount among these will be a call for aggressive containment. This call may involve agitation to initiate social distancing measures, enhance policing of borders between locales affected and not affected, quarantine/isolate those afflicted or exposed, and to close buildings which may have been sites of exposure. In contrast to what happens during a natural outbreak, there may be less resistance from stakeholders when the closure of a site is debated if it is the suspected site of an intentional dissemination of a pathogen.

An immediate demand for post-exposure prophylaxis, which may or may not be necessary, will likely ensue and the possibility of a sudden large spike in cases may leave little time for post-exposure prophylaxis and vaccination plans to be scaled up necessitating the activation of alternate dispensing systems, such as the U.S. Postal Service delivery of antimicrobials [8].

Additionally, if an intentional outbreak occurs, countries may also be less likely to share countermeasures as concerns for domestic populations will take precedence over foreign assistance if stockpiled resources are relatively scarce.

Anxiety and fear amongst the public will tax resources as the "worried well" will present for care or counseling at health care facilities, necessitating triaging to separate true cases (or possible cases) from those at low-risk. During the anthrax attacks in 2001, many emergency departments were subject to people presenting after exposure to a "white powder" seeking treatment for anthrax, and laboratories were tasked with analyzing these suspicious powders [1].

Intense political pressure will mount on those managing an intentional outbreak as their will be pressure to "do something" which could include quarantine measures, identifying culprits, and assessing the ongoing risk of further attacks. This political pressure will necessitate the use of skilled communication strategies that will have to balance the need to identify the perpetrator with informing the public. This strategy may involve withholding crucial information from clinicians and the public in order to not compromise the ongoing forensic investigation.

Because of these differences, intentional outbreaks will likely demand federal government engagement at an early stage, especially if it is large in scale, as local public health departments have minimal surge capacity. Federal engagement could also facilitate utilization of alternate sites of care. In the USA, the CDC and the Federal Bureau of Investigation (FBI) would be important federal assets utilized in an intentional outbreak.

4.4 Considering Engineered Pathogens

The fact that an engineered outbreak has been orchestrated will lead to speculation regarding whether the microbe has been designed to subvert medical countermeasures. Consideration of inserted antimicrobial resistance genes, development of vaccine-escape mutants, enhanced virulence, or enhanced environmental stability will be warranted. These potential design features may justify the use of alternate antimicrobials, less reliance on existing vaccines, more aggressive treatment protocols, and higher levels of decontamination. For example, current guidance for the treatment of anthrax advises the use of two antimicrobials initially to cover the possibility of a resistant strain being involved [5].

4.5 Concomitant Forensic Response

Part of the management of an intentional outbreak will consist of seeking attribution. The forensic investigation will likely proceed in parallel to the epidemiological investigation, but may require more information than is required to clinically manage the outbreak. Whole genome sequencing may be performed in order to definitively identify the outbreak strain with such granularity that it can be determined in which laboratories it has been known to exist. Concerns regarding preserving an intact chain of evidence for future criminal prosecution may be necessary. The FBI's Amerithrax investigation involved microbial forensic techniques that culminated in the identification of genomic mutations and contaminating *Bacillus* species [2].

4.6 A Thinking Enemy

Because an intentional or unnatural outbreak is a clear manifestation of design, when responding to such outbreaks attention to the possibility of novel pathogens and the use of multiple agents will be necessary. Also, if the perpetrators of such an attack are familiar with the response framework of outbreak detection and management, they may have factored the strengths, weaknesses, and processes of that framework into their plans in order to thwart timely detection and mitigation of the outbreak.

4.7 Bioremediation

After an attack, the populace may be justifiably hesitant to re-inhabit a dwelling or site that may have been affected by the outbreak. For example, after the anthrax outbreaks of 2001 several buildings were closed – some for years – and bioremediation costs amounted to hundreds of millions of US dollars [3]. Factoring in bioremediation requirements into the outbreak management from the outset will be necessary in order to prepare stakeholders for future costs and reopening.

4.8 Conclusion

While unnatural or intentional outbreaks are a unique species of outbreaks, many similarities in response plans to natural outbreaks exist and will be relied upon. Areas of departure include anticipating the virulence of the organism, consideration of engineered pathogen strains, coordinating a concomitant forensic investigation, communication strategies, and planning for bioremediation.

References

1. Brannen DE, Stanley SA (2004) Critical issues in bioterrorism preparedness: before and after September 2001. J Public Health Manag Pract 10(4):290–298
2. FBI (2008) Science briefing on the anthrax investigation. 18 August 2008. http://www.fbi.gov/about-us/history/famous-cases/anthrax-amerithrax/science-briefing. Accessed 1 Mar 2011
3. Franco C, Bouri N (2010) Environmental decontamination following a large-scale bioterrorism attack: federal progress and remaining gaps. Biosecur Bioterror 8(2):107–117
4. Hugh-Jones M (2006) Distinguishing between natural and unnatural outbreaks of animal diseases. Revue scientifique et technique (International Office of Epizootics) 25(1):173–186
5. Martin GJ, Friedlander AM (2010) Anthrax as an agent of bioterrorism. In: Mandell GL, Bennett JE, Dolin R (eds) Mandell, Douglas, and Bennett's principles and practice of infectious diseases, 7th edn. Churchill Livingstone, Philadelphia
6. Miller J, Engelberg S, Broad W (2002) Germs. Touchstone, New York
7. Torok TJ, Tauxe RV, Wise RP et al (1997) A large community outbreak of salmonellosis caused by intentional contamination of restaurant salad bars. JAMA 278(5):389–395
8. The White House (2009) Executive order – medical countermeasures following a biological attack. 30 December 2009. http://www.whitehouse.gov/the-press-office/executive-order-medical-countermeasures-following-a-biological-attack. Accessed 1 Mar 2011

Chapter 5
Managing Acute Public Health Events: A World Health Organization Perspective

Catherine Smallwood, Andrew Smith, Nicolas Isla, and Maurizio Barbeschi

Abstract The role of the World Health Organization in managing acute public health events relies on two principles. First of all, strong national public health systems that can maintain active surveillance of diseases and public health events; rapidly investigate detected events; report and assess public health risk; share information; and implement public health control measures. Second, an effective global system that supports disease control programmes to contain public health risks by assessing global trends on a continuous basis and preparing to respond to unexpected and internationally spreading events with a potential for international relevance.

5.1 Introduction

Despite huge advances in our understanding of why diseases occur, how they are transmitted and how effective treatments can be administered, major outbreaks in disease continue to have consequences across the globe. Disease epidemics over the past decade demonstrated that it is not only populations located around the disease source that are at risk from distinct outbreaks but that an outbreak anywhere can affect populations everywhere.

5.2 The World Health Organization's Global Response

The revised International Health Regulations (IHR) (2005) entered into force on 15 June 2007. The revised Regulations provide the international legal framework to identify, assess, communicate, and respond through a collective and

C. Smallwood (✉) • A. Smith • N. Isla • M. Barbeschi
Health Security and Environment, World Health Organization, Geneva, Switzerland
e-mail: smallwoodc@who.int

I. Hunger et al. (eds.), *Biopreparedness and Public Health: Exploring Synergies*, NATO Science for Peace and Security Series A: Chemistry and Biology,
DOI 10.1007/978-94-007-5273-3_5,

all-hazard approach to any threat to public health that has potential for international concern.

The IHR contain rights and obligations for States Parties (and functions for the World Health Organization (WHO)) concerning national and international surveillance; assessment and public health response; health measures applied by States Parties to international travelers, aircraft, ships, motor vehicles and goods; public health at international ports, airports and ground crossings (together referred to as "points of entry"); and many other areas. The revised IHR represent a number of important shifts: from a focus on selected diseases to all public health events of potential international concern; from the control of disease at borders to the containment of disease at source; and from preset measures to adapted responses to events. The revised IHR therefore accommodate natural, environmental, industrial, accidental, or indeed, deliberate threats – they represent an all-hazards approach to public health [8].

5.3 Implementing the Revised IHR

The IHR (2005) defines a risk management process in which member states work with and through WHO in order to collectively manage acute threats to public health. The revised IHR provide obligations for states, including the requirement to have or develop minimum core public health capacities to implement the Regulations effectively. IHR core capacities include legislation and policy; coordination; surveillance; response; preparedness; risk communication; human resources; and laboratory; as well as requirements for points of entry.[1] Key milestones for member states include the assessment of their surveillance and response capacities and the development and implementation of plans of action to ensure that these core capacities are functioning by 2012.

The revised IHR also mandate a key role for WHO in the detection and management of public health events with potential international concern.[2] Under the Regulations, WHO must accurately and rapidly identify and then assess public health risks of potential international concern. If the risk assessment warrants it, WHO must then inform member states of such threats and, upon request, assist affected states with response efforts. Based on the fulfillment of specific criteria, the WHO Director-General may declare an assessed event to be a Public Health Emergency of International Concern (PHEIC) [10].

The capacity to deliver a response under rapidly evolving circumstances is vitally reliant on the engagement and collaboration of all levels of the Organization relating to risk assessment, decision-making, and response processes [9].

[1] As presented by WHO at the IHR Table Top Pilot Workshop, Geneva, 15–17 March 2011.

[2] For the full texts of the IHR (2005) in the six official language versions and related materials, see http://www.who.int/csr/ihr/wha_58_3/en/

5.4 WHO Tools for Alert and Response Operations

WHO implements event-based surveillance to drive the Organization's capacity to detect, assess, inform and respond to public health events of potential international concern. This surveillance harnesses official and unofficial information. Information considered official originates from IHR National Focal Points, national health authorities, other government departments/regulatory authorities, official government websites and publications, WHO regional and country offices, and other UN agencies. Unofficial sources include the news media and electronic public health intelligence feeds (open-source data), and information received from WHO Collaborating Centres, laboratories, academic institutions, and nongovernmental organizations. Such reports are considered to be rumours until they are confirmed as real events by the responsible national authority [10].

The Event Management System (EMS) improves communication and the coordination of international outbreak alert and response [7] and the current web-based EMS meets the needs of the all-hazards approach under the revised IHR. WHO is able to make full use of a single platform for event-based technical and operational information management, and its utility in this regard is demonstrated by the successful roll-out of the EMS to teams at all levels of WHO.[3]

Since April 2000, WHO has supported the development of the Global Outbreak Alert and Response Network (GOARN) to improve international coordination, and provide the operational framework to deliver rapid technical and operational support to member states. This network assists countries with disease control efforts by providing rapid technical support to affected public health systems, investigating events and assessing the risks of emerging epidemic disease threats, and supporting responses that contribute to the sustained containment of epidemic threats.

These activities are supported by dedicated communication, logistics and operation centre teams.

5.5 A "Whole of Society" Approach

The links between health diplomacy, public health, foreign policy and security in achieving global health security have become increasingly clear over the last decade and have been the subject of widespread discussion in various high level fora. A whole of society approach recognizes that collaborations between different sectors contribute to the effective preparedness and management of potential public health risks. Working with all sectors relevant to the identification and response to public health risks of potential international concern has had implications for WHO's work.

[3] For further information, see http://www.who.int/csr/alertresponse/en/

5.6 The Health and Security Interface

WHO has a commitment through its resolutions WHA 54.14 and WHA 55.16 to help member states strengthen their preparedness against biological risks focusing on national and global public health systems. Resolution WHA 55.16 – Response to natural occurrence, accidental release or deliberate use of biological and chemical agents or radionuclear material that affect health – mandates WHO to strengthen global surveillance; help member states strengthen their health systems; issue international guidance on public health measures in response to biological or chemical threats; and examine new tools or mechanisms for modeling possible scenarios for the release of such agents.[4]

In this regard, WHO has a number of ongoing activities at the interface between the health and security sectors. These activities are one part of a broader effort to harness the knowledge and capabilities held within diverse types of organizations and fields in order to enhance WHO's ability to respond to public health risks and emergencies no matter what their origin. In 2011, a Memorandum of Understanding was signed between WHO and the UN Office for Disarmament Affairs to formalize WHO's operational and technical support to the UN Secretary General during investigations of alleged use of biological weapons. The Memorandum of Understanding outlines targets for harmonizing procedures as well as joint training activities and the provision of equipment and expertise.

5.7 Conclusion

WHO believes that strong public health systems will enable populations to withstand and be resilient to the damage caused by public health emergencies, whatever their origin or source. It is with this conviction that WHO will continue to strengthen global and national capacities to counter these risks.

Acknowledgements The authors are, or have been affiliated with the World Health Organization. The authors alone are responsible for the views expressed in this publication and they do not necessarily represent the decisions, policy or views of the World Health Organization.

The authors of this short paper wish to acknowledge and thank several reviewers upon whose work this paper is based. These include members of the Alert and Response Operations team, the Global Capacities, Alert and Response Department, and the Health Security and Environment Cluster, *inter alia*, Paul Cox, Patrick Drury, Angela Merianos, Bruce Plotkin, Faith McLellan and Cathy Roth.

[4] There are other Resolutions that complement the health security framework as provided by the WHA, *i.e.* on Laboratory Biosafety and Biosecurity, Food Safety and INFOSAN etc.

References and Further Reading

1. BWC Meeting of the States Parties (2010) Synthesis of considerations, lessons, perspectives, recommendations, conclusions and proposals drawn from the presentations, statements, working papers and interventions on the topic under discussion at the Meeting of Experts. Meeting of the States Parties to the BWC, Geneva, 6–10 December 2010
2. International Air Transport Association (2011) Fact sheet: IATA, Geneva. http://www.iata.org/pressroom/facts_figures/fact_sheets/Documents/Industry-Facts-March-2011.pdf
3. WHO (2001) A framework for global outbreak alert and response, Geneva. http://www.who.int/csr/resources/publications/surveillance/WHO_CDS_CSR_2000_2/en/
4. WHO (2004) Globalization and infectious diseases: a review of the linkages. Social, Economic, and Behavioural Research. Special Topics No. 3, Geneva. http://apps.who.int/tdr/svc/publications/tdr-research-publications/globalization-infectious-diseases
5. WHO (2005) Outbreak communication: Best practices for communicating with the public during an outbreak. Report of the WHO Expert Consultation on Outbreak Communications held in Singapore, 21–23 September 2004, Geneva. http://www.who.int/csr/resources/publications/WHO_CDS_2005_32/en/index.html
6. WHO Western Pacific Regional Office (2006) SARS: How a global epidemic was stopped. WHO, Manila
7. WHO (2006) Openness is key in fight against disease outbreaks. Bulletin of the World Health Organization. October 2006. vol 84(10). Geneva. http://www.who.int/bulletin/volumes/84/10/news.pdf
8. WHO (2007) A safer future: global public health security in the 21st century. The World Health Report 2007, Geneva. http://www.who.int/whr/2007/en/index.html
9. WHO (2008a), Best practices for WHO epidemic alert and response, Geneva. http://www.who.int/csr/Best_Practices.pdf
10. WHO (2008b) WHO event management for international public health security: operational procedures, Geneva. http://www.who.int/csr/resources/publications/WHO_HSE_EPR_ARO_2008_1/en/index.html
11. WHO (2011) IHR core capacity monitoring framework: checklist and indicators for monitoring progress in the development of IHR core capacities in States Parties, February 2011, Geneva. http://www.who.int/ihr/IHR_Monitoring_Framework_Checklist_and_Indicators.pdf

Chapter 6
Public Health in South-Eastern Europe – Exploring Synergies

Dorit Nitzan Kaluski and Maria Ruseva

Abstract In the past decade countries in the South-eastern Europe Health Network (SEEHN) have been making big strides to reform their health systems. The SEEHN has been providing a platform to share experiences and opening doors to resources, partnerships, technical capacity and political commitment. The ability of health systems to prevent, react, mitigate and recover from emergencies and crises is a visible indicator for the functionality of the health systems. In some of the health systems in the SEEHN there are still gaps that do not allow for a smooth and a seamless ability to respond to such demanding needs. Sometimes, parts of the populations are not accessible to the health services, and in many the public health services do not have sufficient finances and capacity to carry their tasks. Potential synergies between public health services and other arms of the health systems and beyond should be strengthened in SEEHN Member States. The WHO agenda for public health, health system strengthening and Health in All Policies continue to bring together the know-how, the ideology, partnerships, resource generation and the platform for subsequent policy development and implementation.

6.1 Background

In the period before 1990 the public health services in South-eastern Europe (SEE) were organized largely according to the highly centralized models (e.g. Semashko Model). Accordingly, the Public Health Institutes had to fulfill the

D.N. Kaluski (✉)
WHO Country Office in Serbia, Public Health Services for South-eastern Europe,
WHO Regional Office for Europe, Belgrade, Serbia
e-mail: dnk@who.org.rs

M. Ruseva
Public Health Services, WHO Regional Office for Europe, Copenhagen, Denmark
e-mail: mah@euro.who.int

I. Hunger et al. (eds.), *Biopreparedness and Public Health: Exploring Synergies*,
NATO Science for Peace and Security Series A: Chemistry and Biology,
DOI 10.1007/978-94-007-5273-3_6,

following tasks: control of communicable diseases; sanitary-hygienic inspections and overall control of suspected hazards and health education. Typically, each Public Health Institute (PHI) comprised the following units: environmental health; occupational health; nutrition and food hygiene; child and adolescent health; and communicable disease control (e.g. epidemiology and microbiology).

At the turn of the 1990s, with the break-up of Yugoslavia and the turmoil that lasted more than a decade, the countries in the SEE were faced with a stark reality: economic deterioration, political instability, social turmoil and stagnation. The conflict led to a high number of internally displaced people (IDPs), refugees, and a vast migration among the professionals. The socio-economic gaps and poverty rates increased. Soon after the crisis, the rapid shift from a planned to a market economy resulted in health systems reforms that many times left the public health services (PHS) in the margins of the health and social systems, without the support needed to implement their functions.

In September 2000, representatives from 189 countries adopted the Millennium Development Goals (MDGs), a series of time-limited commitments to reduce poverty and promote human development. At the heart of these commitments were the goals to tackle urgent public health issues by the target date of 2015. The challenges for SEE Member States to not only restore their public health systems to the pre-1990s situation, but rather to rapidly develop health systems that would match their needs have been recognized by the WHO European Region.

6.2 WHO Support to SEE During the Decade of Turmoil

WHO coordinated health activities and provided technical assistance to the SEE countries during the decade of turmoil. It ensured an orientation inline with the national health policies, health reform trends and international standards. WHO implemented humanitarian programmes in the former Yugoslavia; carried out needs monitoring; advocacy with donors; assistance to the most vulnerable; linking humanitarian programmes with the much needed humanitarian assistance and contributed to the UN Consolidated Appeals (CAPs). At that time, a bottom-up approach was used through institutional, social grass root partnerships between institutions and civil societies.

Following are some examples: in the UN Administered Province of Kosovo, WHO contributed to the rehabilitation of the health system in cooperation with the UN Mission to Kosovo (UNMIK), developed health policy guidelines with coordination with organizations working in the health arena, especially those in primary and public health services, including disease control, environmental health, community-based mental health programmes and support to mother and child health services. WHO facilitated the accessibility of refugees to health services and provided technical support to the Ministry of Health of the Former Yugoslav Republic of Macedonia. In Croatia, local authorities – assisted by WHO – established surveillance systems that were valuable for planning interventions. Using the ATLAS, the WHO worked with the authorities in Bosnia and Herzegovina to engage in mental health and the elderly. The PRINT Project is an example of an action directed at populations hit by the consequences of war and for the repatriation and reinsertion of refugees and displaced populations.

During that period, partners and WHO worked in SEE to support the peace process and renewal of social development; to allow communities to take an active part in the rehabilitation process and peaceful coexistence and solidarity; and to promote solidarity for the most vulnerable groups. In this regard a special attention was given to IDPs, refugees and returnees, people who suffered from post-traumatic stress disorder and mental health diseases, and the disabled, wounded and injured.

6.3 SEE Health Network

In 1999, the international community established the Stability Pact for SEE as a conflict-prevention and reconstruction process in the region. In 2001, a health component, SEE Health Network (SEEHN), was added to the Pact's Social Cohesion Initiative, to bring people together across borders to improve health in the whole region [5]. SEEHN has received continuous political, technical and financial support from 11 partner countries (Belgium, France, Greece, Hungary, Italy, Netherlands, Norway, Slovenia, Sweden, Switzerland and the United Kingdom) and five international organizations.

SEEHN is a political and institutional forum set up by the governments of Albania, Bosnia and Herzegovina, Bulgaria, Croatia, Montenegro, the Republic of Moldova, Romania, Serbia, and the Former Yugoslav Republic of Macedonia to promote peace, reconciliation and health in the region. WHO Regional Office for Europe has been lending technical support to SEEHN's various health projects, after having supplied its secretariat, along with the Council of Europe, from 2001 to 2012.

On 1 January 2010, the SEEHN took over ownership over the regional cooperation for health and development under the auspices of the Regional Cooperation Council (RCC) and the SEE Regional Cooperation Process. RCC's main purpose is to provide leadership and to sustain ownership by the nine countries of regional cooperation and the concerted health development action launched in 2001 with the Dubrovnik Pledge [1] maintained through the 2005 Skopje Pledge [2], the 2009 Memorandum of Understanding, and the 2011 Banja Luka Pledge [3].

For more than a decade, SEEHN has been the undisputed vehicle of health development in the areas of mental health, communicable diseases, food safety and nutrition, blood safety, tobacco control, information systems, maternal and neonatal health, public health services and health systems.

The achievements of the network can be categorized:

1. Contribution to the peace building and stabilization process – through creating a wide network of experts at all levels as well as of political representatives:
   - Over 250 people are contributing to the cooperation.
   - Partnerships with several political and international organizations including the European Union, Regional Cooperation Council, Northern Dimension Partnership for Public Health and Social Well-Being.

2. Development, improvement and alignment of health policies and legislation with WHO conventions and regulation and European legislation, including national strategies and work-plans:

   - Support to the implementation of the IHRs, surveillance of communicable diseases.
   - Ratification of the FCTC and approval of tobacco control laws.
   - Orienting health strategy of caring for mental health and disabled children at community level.
   - Re-orienting the former psychiatric care towards de-institutionalization and care in the community with respect to human rights of people with mental disabilities; establishment of ten Community Mental Health Centres in the nine countries with a catchment area on over one million citizens.
   - Approval of food safety laws and regulations in support of consumer protection.
   - Developing and updating national strategies for improving maternal and neonatal health.

3. Capacity-building through experience exchange and training for experts of nine technical areas at different levels:
   - Numerous project meetings at regional and country level on all projects.
   - Ten regional publications on the thematic areas of work.
   - Regional and national level assessments.

4. A strong feeling of ownership, trust and confidence was attained by the countries as a result of the delegation and empowerment principles applied, which led to their increased responsibility for and participation in various roles and structures in the project.
5. Spirit of openness, transparency and accountability in both the dialogue and actions was developed and sustained which increased trust and confidence.
6. Establishment of strong partnerships among the nine SEE countries on one side and with six donor and neighboring countries on the other

6.4 SEEHN Public Health Services Project

The Skopje Pledge (mentioned above) commits the members of the SEEHN to improve the health systems of the SEE countries to secure universal access to high-quality PHS, and thus the PHS Project became one of the nine regional projects of the SEEHN. The SEEHN has overseen its implementation with the technical support of the WHO Regional Office for Europe, financial support of the Council of Europe Development Bank (CEB) and with the in-kind support of the Department of Health for England [6].

The evaluation of PHS in SEE countries and the production of national and regional reports on PHS was a key undertaking of the SEEHN. The evaluation formed the first component of the PHS project "Strengthening public health capacity and services".

6.5 Evaluation of the Public Health Services in SEE

The evaluation of PHS was carried out by the SEEHN and was aimed at assessing their "essential public health operations". The essential public health operations that were used in the evaluation include:

1. Surveillance and assessment of the population's health and well-being;
2. Identifying health problems and health hazards in the community;
3. Preparedness and planning for public health emergencies;
4. Health protection (environmental, occupational, food safety and others);
5. Disease prevention;
6. Health promotion;
7. Evaluation of quality and effectiveness of personal and community health services;
8. Assuring a competent public health and personal health care workforce.

6.6 Key Findings

6.6.1 SEE Stewardship of Public Health

Among the strengths of PHS in SEE one can note the general stance for universal health coverage and equal access to services as defined in the laws. Also, there are legal frameworks for public health, defined packages of services, established PHIs and well-established processes for policy formation and strategy development. In general, there is a positive role of international partners and NGOs, with strong broader international context and framework that can be seen by the many signed charters and agreements in the area of public health. Population health surveillance systems are well established, in most places.

However, in most of the member states there is insufficient intersectorial collaboration in many areas, including intersectorial assessment of policies, strategies and programmes. Usually, there is no comprehensive use of social determinants of health (SDH) to inform policy. This is partly due to lack of disaggregated data. Moreover, routine data on the prevalence of certain risk factors is inadequate. Even in cases where the policy-legal level are sufficient, there might be inadequate implementation of legislation and regulations. Survey findings are used neither sufficiently nor systematically in the development of policy. Additional information gathering is needed to support policy design.

6.6.2 Public Health Service Delivery

In all SEE countries there is a PHI network, with its well defined surveillance systems and organized institutional networks for control of communicable diseases.

In principle, robust crisis management arrangements should be in place. In most of the countries there are effective and comprehensive vaccination programmes and coverage, at least for the registered population. There are food safety control systems in place throughout most of the region, as well as established procedures for the control of air, water and sanitation. A significant attention is given to environmental protection issues.

Nevertheless, there is insufficient coordination and seamless division of authority, responsibility and accountability; the role for primary health care and PHS not clearly defined. SDH are not reflected or incorporated into services and Health in All Policies is not fully in place.

In many of the SEE countries, some of the residents do not have access to health services because they do not have health cards, which could be due to lack of identity cards, lack of employment or inability to register as unemployed, lack of pension, or other. In some countries, these people have access only to emergency services, but not to primary care or public health services.

6.6.3 *Financing of the PHS*

Most of the funding for core public health services is provided directly by the state. In most countries, there is a system of mandatory health insurance, with defined packages of services, at least for those with health cards.

In general, the funds for the public health system are not sufficient. In some countries the PHS "sell services" for funds, an issue that might be at risk for conflict of interest.

Following are a few examples:

1. Albania – The IPH and the Veterinary Institute carry out an Integrated Surveillance System of Infectious Diseases (AISSID). The IHR is under the responsibility of the respective technical health personnel throughout the country. National immunization programmes are provided only for children up to 14 years of age. The Ministry of Health has designated technical staff responsible for Disaster Planning and Response (DPR).
2. Bosnia and Herzegovina – Under Federal Law on Health Care, the Federal Public Health Institute (FPHI) provides a system for monitoring public health, analyzing health trends and combating disease. At the municipal level, PHS are mainly responsible for hygienic-epidemiologic services. At the cantonal level ten PHIs monitor the epidemiological situation and offer expert advice to tackle epidemics. The FPHI coordinates the work of the cantonal public health institutes. The system is under-resourced, particularly in the area of identifying infectious agents. Laws covering water and air quality were adopted in 2003, but are not fully implemented. Hazardous waste and medical waste are particularly critical and represent one of the most serious threats to health. The Federal Administration for Civil Protection is responsible for implementation of the Law on Disaster Preparedness and

Response (2003), which includes a provision on public health. Vaccination is mandatory for children and against rabies. The laws on water and air protection and the management of non-radioactive waste are in line with EU policy. A National Environmental Action Plan (NEAP) and a National Environmental Health Action Plan (NEHAP) are in place.

3. Bulgaria – A medical specialist who first detects an outbreak is required by law to report it to the 28 Regional Health Inspectorates (RHI), which communicate the information to the Ministry of Health and to the National Centre for Infections and Parasitic Diseases (NCIPD). General practitioners, school-based medical specialists, child establishments, specialized health institutions and RHI register diagnosed communicable diseases in a special log. A national plan for crisis management includes organization of medical care for victims: sorting, evacuation, treatment, interaction between medical and non-medical personnel and optimal use of resources. Each medical institution has a detailed emergency plan also for bio-hazards. Detection of outbreaks includes regulations for the registration and control of nosocomial infections. In-hospital antibiotic resistance is monitored nationally.
4. Croatia – The three-tier system for surveillance and detection of communicable diseases is coordinated centrally and involves 21 PHIs and 113 first-level epidemiology units. Notification of infectious diseases is mandatory through a 24/7 early warning system. Daily, weekly and monthly monitoring and analyses of communicable disease reports occurs at all three levels.
5. Montenegro – IPH surveillance of communicable diseases is carried out by local health centres. There is a compulsory reporting system on morbidity and mortality for 75 communicable diseases. The Ministry of Interior has adopted a strategy for emergency situations and response. It includes natural disasters, chemical and radiological hazards, outbreaks and bioterrorism. There is no emergency plan that defines organizational responsibilities, communication and information networks, and clearly outlines alert and evacuation protocols. The IPH does not have a roster of personnel with the technical expertise to respond to potential biological, chemical, or radiological public health emergencies.
6. Moldova – Preparedness for health and other emergencies is covered by the law. The Service for Civil Protection and Extraordinary Situations provides overall crisis management. A special provision requires the identification and control of public health threats from factors such as pollution, radioactivity, toxins and biological agents. Emergency response is also the responsibility of the Governmental National Emergency Commission and territorial commissions. A mandatory surveillance and reporting system for infectious diseases operates at national, regional and community level. The Ministry of Health maintains 24/7 communication channels to issue alerts about epidemics of infectious diseases. Local commissions coordinate an intersectorial response. The teams include epidemiologists and experts on food, air and water safety, toxicology and radiology. Clinicians and laboratory support are provided by the National Scientific and Practical Centre for Preventive Medicine and other relevant institutions. The Ministry of Health does not have a crisis management unit and has no defined

budget for emergency preparedness. There is a need for more centrally coordinated technical-level cooperation between health agencies, for more comprehensive training in crisis management, and for a greater emphasis on emergency medical services (EMS) and emergency response.

7. Romania – Surveillance system for detecting outbreaks is under the responsibility of the Ministry of Health/Public Health Authority, National Centre for Communicable Disease Prevention and Control (NCCDPC), National Institute of Research and Development for Microbiology and Immunology "Cantacuzino" (NIRDMI-C) and include the epidemiological departments of the four regional institutes in Bucharest, Cluj, Iasi and Timisoara, the district health authorities (DHAs) and specialist hospitals, and physicians. The national laboratory is participating in the national surveillance programme for neuro-invasive West-Nile infections. On request, the national reference laboratory provides services for hemorrhagic fevers (e.g. hemorrhagic fever with renal syndrome) and tick-borne encephalitis. There is also capacity for confirming other vector-borne diseases, such as Lyme disease, Rickettsia conorii and Coxiella burnetii. The National Laboratory for Parasitic Diseases at the NIRDMI-C is a reference laboratory for malaria. The Entomology National Reference Laboratory at the NIRDMI-C participates in the European Commission's EDEN (Emerging Diseases in a Changing European Environment) research project. At the national level it is involved in developing surveillance methodologies for vector- and animal-borne diseases. It performs susceptibility tests for vector-borne diseases and monitors the circulation of vector-borne disease pathogens (in vectors and/or animals).
8. Serbia – The National Institute of Public Health and 23 IPHs coordinate public health at the central and regional level. The IPHs function in two modalities: "institut za javno zdravlje" function in cities where there is a medical faculty (e.g. Belgrade, Novi Sad, Kragujevac, and Nis). These institutes provide teaching for medical students, while the institutes in other districts are called "zavod". One of the IPHs is located in Kosovo (in accordance with UN Security Council resolution 1244 (1999)) and is serving the Serbs that reside in the Mitrovica area and in the Serbian enclaves. All IPHs have their own web-sites. Health related data is collected by the local IPH and are transferred to the National IPH. According to the Health Care Law each of the IPH is comprised of six centres and two departments (i.e. Health Promotion Centre, Disease Control and Prevention Centre, Centre for Hygiene and Medical Ecology, Centre for Microbiology, Centre for Informatics and Biostatistics , Centre for Health Planning, Department for Health Care Organization, and Department for Financing and Legal Issues). It also includes administrative and technical support. IPHs functions are defined by the Law: monitoring, evaluation and analysis of the health status of the population; monitoring and assessment of burden of diseases and risk factors; suggestion of elements to health policy, plans and programmes with measures and activities to promote the health of the population, health education and training of the population; assessment of efficiency, availability and quality of health services, human resource for health system planning and development; development of integrated health information system; public health research; and development of

partnerships with communities, governmental and non-governmental organizations. There is no activity aimed at emergencies and crises management. In reality, the IPHs are under-funded and are unable to perform their full activities as requested by the Law and the health reform. A third of their funds is provided by the Ministry of Health. These funds are given for specific programmes or projects. About a third is provided by the National Health Insurance Fund to cover for reporting on health system performance activities, while the IPHs have to obtain the rest from selling their services to the private sector for the assessment of water and air quality and for the provision of sanitary inspection.

9. The Former Yugoslav Republic of Macedonia – Physicians are required by law to report immediately any suspected cases, or carriers, of communicable diseases, according to the Communicable Diseases List, suspected outbreaks, cases of nosocomial infection, cases of post-vaccination complications, and each bite or injury by an animal infected or suspected of having rabies. The Law on Crisis Management has established a system to anticipate and manage crises caused by disasters and epidemics, or other non-military events that imperil public health and property. The Centre for Crisis Management analyses all data relating to potential crises, such as outbreaks of communicable diseases, bioterrorism, chemical and radiological hazards and natural disasters.

6.7 Conclusion

Prevention of crises and emergencies, preparedness and response require that all functions of health systems (e.g. stewardship, resource generation, financing and service delivery) are coordinated and are driven by the guiding principles of equity, social justice, social participation and inter-sectorial collaboration.

The World Health Organization Regional Office for Europe commitment to the provision of equitable good-quality health services and for building strong health systems has been shared with the SEEHN. Attention has been given to vulnerable populations and marginalized communities to mitigate those factors that entwine poverty, morbidity and mortality.

Ministries of Health could benefit from strengthening their functions and to enable them to lead and to steer on a horizontal, cross-cutting, whole policy, multi-tiered response, within the country and with intersectorial partners [4].

References

1. SEEHN (2001) South-eastern Europe Health Network, The Dubrovnik Pledge, Meeting the health needs of vulnerable populations in South East Europe, Dubrovnik, Croatia, 2 September 2001. http://www.euro.who.int/__data/assets/pdf_file/0009/99738/e94525.pdf
2. SEEHN (2005) South-eastern Europe Health Network, The Skopje Pledge, Health and economic development in South-eastern Europe, Skopje, Former Yugoslav Republic of Macedonia, 15 November 2005. http://www.euro.who.int/__data/assets/pdf_file/0005/99743/E88513.pdf

3. SEEHN (2011) South-eastern Europe Health Network, The Banja Luka Pledge, Health in all policies in South-eastern Europe: A shared goal and responsibility, Banja Luka, Bosnia and Herzegovina, 13–14 October 2011. http://www.euro.who.int/__data/assets/pdf_file/0020/152471/e95832.pdf
4. WHO (2009) Maximizing positive synergies between health systems and global health initiatives. http://www.who.int/healthsystems/New-approach-leaflet-ENv2-p4p.pdf
5. WHO Regional Office for Europe (2011) South-eastern Europe Health Network. http://www.euro.who.int/stabilitypact/network/20040611_1
6. WHO Regional Office for Europe, Council of Europe Development Bank (2009) Evaluation of public health services in South-eastern Europe. http://www.euro.who.int/__data/assets/pdf_file/0016/125206/e94398.pdf

Chapter 7
Health Security and Disease Detection in the European Union

Massimo Ciotti

Abstract In a globalised world, national and international institutions in charge of health security can no longer only rely on traditional disease reporting mechanisms, not designed to recognise emergence of new hazards. New approaches are developing to improve the capacity of surveillance systems in detecting previously unknown threats. More recently, surveillance institutions have been actively searching for information about health threats using internet scanning tools, email distribution lists or networks that complement the early warning function of routine surveillance systems. Since its foundation, ECDC has developed an epidemic intelligence framework that encompasses all activities related to early identification of potential health hazards, their verification, assessment and investigation, in order to recommend public health control measures. Since June 2005, about 900 threats have been monitored by ECDC. Several threats made it necessary to develop formal risk assessments or to dispatch ECDC experts to outbreak areas. Examples of recent events, identified through the epidemic intelligence activity, are presented to illustrate the course of action from threat detection through risk management in Europe.

7.1 Introduction

During the last decades public health scientists have been confronted with the detection, assessment and management of a number of threats with increasing risk of spreading internationally. Globalization of food and product trade, as well as the steady increase of worldwide travel, contributes to an increasing awareness of global communicable disease threats and to the need for preparing the public health

---

M. Ciotti (✉)
Public Health Capacity and Communication Unit,
European Centre for Disease Prevention and Control, Stockholm, Sweden
e-mail: massimo.ciotti@ecdc.europa.eu

I. Hunger et al. (eds.), *Biopreparedness and Public Health: Exploring Synergies*,
NATO Science for Peace and Security Series A: Chemistry and Biology,
DOI 10.1007/978-94-007-5273-3_7,

systems to respond to unexpected epidemics. The possibility of bioterrorist attacks in recent years has reinforced the rationale for a broader approach to public health security.

7.2 European Union Policies and Activities

The European Union (EU) and its 27 member states will continue facing considerable challenges regarding communicable disease in the years to come, including the threat of the release of man-made biological agents at a small or large scale.

Public health protection, according to the current EU legislation, is mostly a shared competence of the EU institutions and the member states. Countries in the EU are at different stages of preparedness to respond to major threats, including those originated by the intentional release of biological agents. The differences in completion of national plans to counter bioterrorism are partly due to the significant variance in the perception of threat in the EU member states [2] as well as to different levels of competence within the governmental structures in charge of security.

The risk of international spread of an infectious disease was considered a priority in the EU already in 1996. Provisions were developed to ensure open communication channels between the relevant authorities; a list of communicable diseases was agreed upon, which were to be under surveillance by all member states, and common case definitions for these diseases were developed [5].

After the September 11th terrorist aggression in the USA and the later anthrax attacks, it became clearer that public health and infectious diseases should be considered and treated as a strategic national priority. The EU responded to these challenges by creating the Health Security Committee (HSC) under the directorate for public health, with the mandate to coordinate and complement national measures in the area of health security. Strategic work plans were then developed to guide the actions of the committee [12]. The European Commission worked on the adopted relevant Health Security Programme of co-operation on preparedness and response against biological and chemical threats, creating also mechanisms of communication during health security crises [3, 23]. The appearance of a global threat, such as the emergence of SARS in 2002, and the need of scientific coordination of complex assessment of threats affecting more than one country, elicited the decision of the EU in 2004 to create the European Centre for Disease Prevention and Control (ECDC) with the mandate of strengthening the preparedness and response against health threats in the EU [21].

7.3 EU Crisis Response Mechanisms

The Treaty on the Functioning of the European Union [24], entered into force on 1 December 2009, contains several references to the role of institutions, their coordination with member states and international partners, and the sharing of resources, all based on the principle of solidarity in response to major crises. Article 168 specifically deals with public health in stating that a "high level of human health protection shall be ensured in the definition and implementation of all Union policies and activities", and that "Community action shall be directed towards improving public health, preventing human illness and diseases, and obviating sources of danger to human health" by "encouraging cooperation between the member States" and "lending support to their action". Actions to fight against major health threats also include "monitoring, early warning of and combating of cross-border health threats".

The political coordination of crises of relevance to the EU is performed through the Emergency and Crisis Coordination Arrangements (CCA) of the Council and the European Commission [6]. Its functions are to support the political coordination, to exchange information among decision-makers, and to test procedures through regular simulation exercises (e.g. a 2010 exercise scenario of a bio-attack, testing arrangements to ensure quick and adequate crisis response/information flow and identify policy gaps). Other mechanisms, with legal and financial instruments, also exist. One is the Monitoring and Information Centre (MIC) for EU civil protection (DG ECHO) with the aim to pool and deploy immediate civil protection and medical assistance including the mobilisation of pre-registered CBRN modules, from member states to countries affected by major emergencies–inside and outside the EU [18].

In the public health area, the Health Security Committee (HSC), created by a Council decision in 2001, is a decision-making body supporting the EU Commission on preparedness planning and crisis response management in health emergencies. Its mandate is currently under review and since 2007 includes CBRN, generic preparedness, and pandemic influenza. The HSC is composed of high level representatives of the EU Health Ministers and the European Commission. A proposal for a decision of the European Parliament and of the Council [4] has been launched in 2011 with the aim to streamline and strengthen the EU capacities and structures for responding to serious cross-border threats to health, including the formalization of the HSC.

Generally, the assessment and the management aspects of crises are distinct responsibilities. As far as public health is concerned, the national public health institute of a member state, where existent, is in charge of risk assessment, including disease surveillance activities and outbreak investigation. Management aspects are usually handled by the Ministry of Health, which is responsible for prevention and control measures. These two institutions work closely together. Even though this is the most common model, this structure may vary between countries. At EU level, the European Commission is responsible for all management aspects of infectious diseases, whereas the ECDC is in charge of the assessment of public health threats and the provision of technical expertise to member states. In the area of crisis management, the European Commission and the specialised agencies of the EU maintain and support a number of monitoring and alert systems for threat detection, risk assessment, rapid alert and risk management (Table 7.1) and platforms for crisis management, all of which provide means for information exchange and dissemination, as well as coordination with member states and international organizations (Table 7.2).

Table 7.1 EU rapid alert and notification systems for crisis management

Function	Rapid alert and notification system	Description of system	Legal basis
All crises	ARGUS	Internal communication network for concerned DG services during crisis situations	2005/662/EC
		Some Community rapid alert and notification systems feed into ARGUS	2006/25/EC
General civil protection	CECIS (Common Emergency Communication and Information System)	Web-based, 24/7, communication and information sharing between the Monitoring and Information Centre of DG ECHO (Civil Protection) and designated contact points in the EU member states	2001/792/EC
		Is used to: send and receive alerts, provide details of assistance required, to make offers to help, and to provide overview of ongoing emergency in an online logbook	2007/162/EC
Radiological emergencies and nuclear accidents	ECURIE (European Community Urgent Radiological Information Exchange)	Web-based, 24/7, radiological emergency notification and subsequent information (urgent messages) exchange system between contact points in the participating countries	87/600/Euratom
Food and feed emergencies	ADNS (Animal Disease Notification System)	Notification system on contagious animal disease outbreaks	2004/216/EC
Food and feed emergencies	RASFF (Rapid Alert System for Food and Feed)	Rapid alert system for food and feed to exchange information in cases where risk to human health is identified in food or feed products and measures have to be taken	2002/178/EC
Communicable diseases	EWRS (Early Warning and Response System)	Early warning and response system to alert public health authorities in the EU member states and the European Commission on outbreaks of communicable diseases (with restricted access)	2000/57/EC

Biological and chemical threats	RAS-BICHAT (Rapid Alert System on Biological and Chemical Agent Attack Taskforce)	Web-based rapid alert system used for exchanging information on health threats due to deliberate release of chemical, biological and radio-nuclear agents Used for notification of threats, exchange of information and coordination of measures among partners	1998/2119/EC
Chemical threats	RAS-CHEM (Rapid Alert System for Chemical Incidents)	Rapid alert system linking the various poison centres of the EU and the Ministries of Health for the exchange of information on incidents including chemical agents relevant to terrorism and other events leading to release of chemicals, and for the consultation and coordination of counter-measures	1998/2119/EC
Plant or plant product emergencies	EUROPHYT (European Network of Plant Health Information Systems) Phytosanitary network	Rapid exchange of intercepted information Provides database for relevant information on interceptions of harmful organisms or prohibited plants and plant products, originating in EU or 3rd countries Enables dissemination, analysis of information related to interceptions Notifies national plant protection organization of country of origin in cases of interceptions in 3rd countries	2000/29/EC
Non-food consumer emergencies	RAPEX (Rapid Alert System for Non-Food Consumer Products)	Provides rapid exchange of information on measures taken by national authorities and/or product distributers on non-food consumer products posing a serious risk to health and safety of consumers	2001/95/EC
Economic security/Protection of EU budget	AFIS (Anti Fraud Information System)	Rapid exchange of information on fraud between the European Commission and the competent authorities in the EU member states	Mutual Assistance Regulation (515/97)

(continued)

Table 7.1 (continued)

Function	Rapid alert and notification system	Description of system	Legal basis
Energy and transport security	CIWIN (Critical Infrastructure Warning Information Network)	Information exchange tool on critical infra-structure (energy and transport networks) through designated contact points in the EU; member states inform the European Commission about threats, risks and vulnerabilities in specific critical infrastructure sectors	COM (2008) 676
Socio-political conflicts/ Humanitarian natural disasters	TARÎQA	Rapid alert system for political and humanitarian crises, enabling the alerting of political and humanitarian crises which appear in the media	2006/1717/EC
	RELEX Crisis Platform	Open source intelligence platform developed by the European Commission's Directorate-General for External Relations. It is a heuristic tool – supported by a multimedia content database – that facilitates search, investigation, analysis and discovery	

Table 7.2 Commission information exchange/dissemination/coordination platforms for crisis management

Function	Coordination platform	Description of system	Legal basis
General civil protection	CECIS (Common Emergency and Information System)	Web-based, 24/7, Communication and information sharing between the MIC and designated contact points in the EU member states	2001/792/EC
		Is used to send and receive alerts, provide details of assistance required, to make offers to help, and to provide overview of ongoing emergency in an online logbook	2007/162/EC
Radiological emergencies and nuclear accidents	ECURIE (European Community Urgent Radiological Information Exchange)	24/7 web-based radiological emergency notification and subsequent information (urgent messages) exchange system between contact points in the participating countries	87/600/Euratom
	EURODEP (European Radiological Data Exchange Platform)	Network/platform for daily and emergency (hourly) exchange of automatic monitoring data from European radiological monitoring networks (4,500 stations)	87/600/Euratom
	ENSEMBLE (Platform for model evaluation and ensemble analysis of atmospheric chemistry transport and dispersion models)	Coordination platform to support emergency management and decision-making in relation to long range atmospheric dispersion modeling	87/600/Euratom
		Under emergency conditions, the system allows for immediate and direct comparison amongst atmospheric dispersion modeling results, and subsequently allows to determine the level of consensus in forecasting the evolution of the dispersing cloud	
		The ENSEMBLE network is composed of meteorological centres in 20 countries, mainly in Europe but also Canada, Japan and USA	

(continued)

Table 7.2 (continued)

Function	Coordination platform	Description of system	Legal basis
Diseases and health emergencies	HEDIS (Health Emergency and Diseases Information System)	For information exchange and awareness during infectious outbreaks and health emergencies and response phases	2000/57/EC
		Logbook of actions taken, document repository, database of models, maps of events	
	TeSsy (The European Surveillance System) (ECDC)	Integrated European communicable disease surveillance system	851/2004/EC
	EPIS (Epidemic Intelligence System) (ECDC)	Epidemic intelligence portal for outbreak detection, risk assessment, outbreak investigation and control measures at EU level	851/2004/EC
Plant or plant product emergencies	EUROPHYT (Phytosanitary network)	Rapid exchange of intercepted information	2000/29/EC
		Provides database for relevant information on interceptions of harmful organisms or prohibited plants and plant products, originating in EU or third countries	
		Enables dissemination, analysis of information related to interceptions	
		Notifies national plant protection organization of country of origin in cases of interceptions in third countries	
Socio-political conflicts/ Humanitarian disasters	KREIOS (Information exchange between Situation Centres)	24/7 web-based platform for unique information exchange during crisis and non-crisis times	2006/1717/EC
Border management	Information sharing and coordination systems platforms	Information sharing platform	2007/2004/ (26.10.2004, OJ L 349/ 25.11.2004) EC
		FIS (FRONTEX Information System)	
		CRATE, a system for the management of the pooled technical equipment and members of the Rapid Pool	

The role and mandate of the ECDC regarding health threats is limited to risk monitoring, assessment and communication. In situations where a health threat affects more than one member state and a multi-country response is needed, public health measures are taken with joint efforts by the European Commission and the national authorities. The implementation of public health measures is the responsibility of member states according to their jurisdictional organisation. The role of an EU agency, such as the ECDC, is to provide expertise and technical support to risk managers when called on to do so. This can include evidence-based risk assessment and "hands on" support in investigating outbreaks.

7.4 A Broader Public Health Stance

A common thread connects all preparedness and response processes and this is represented by an "all-hazards" outlook in the preparedness of the public health sector. A broad understanding of the problem makes it easier to focus on synergies instead of trade-offs between the partners and sectors involved. Currently the ECDC works following a matrix model which combines its four core vertical functions (surveillance, scientific advice, preparedness and response, and health communication) with programmes focused on priority areas of communicable diseases. This structure also facilitates the integration of the deliberate release perspective in the current ECDC work.

The most important differentiating factor in countering an incident of deliberate release as opposed to a naturally occurring epidemic is the need for collaboration with the security sector and the law enforcement authorities. In response to an incident of deliberate release, public health services continue to operate their surveillance systems and analyse case findings, investigate and test samples in diagnostic laboratories, give guidance for managing patients and propose public health measures for the control of the outbreak as in any other infectious disease emergency. In their relationship with security sector and law enforcement authorities, public health services stress the importance of keeping public health high on the agenda in cases of a deliberate release of biological agents. However, in response to a health crisis resulting from a deliberate release of a biological agent, EU coordination is faced with two contradicting forces in the communication with the member states: on the one hand some member states would be requesting urgent advice, guidance and possibly assistance, while on the other hand there will be marked reluctance by the security sector to discuss sensitive information.

Yet, public health systems can respond rapidly with effective containment measures only when the best evidence-based options are supported by early warnings and plausible information on the source of the outbreak, its characteristics, and the extent of its public health impact. Official notifications, as in routine surveillance, often are insufficient, belated and subject to a lengthy clearance, and are of little help when a rapid and effective response is necessary.

7.5 Early Detection of Disease Outbreaks

Modern technologies, mainly related to the development of information technology, with the internet being the backbone of it, are rapidly changing the way scientists and public health officials access health information. Online media, scientific fora and direct electronic communication are increasingly supplanting traditional reporting mechanisms through the various levels of public health administration. Health authorities are no longer in full control of an environment that puts journalists, politicians and the general public in direct contact with raw data.

This new information environment contributed to the revision of the International Health Regulations that was approved during the 2005 World Health Assembly. Member states of the World Health Organization (WHO) are legally bound to both notify cases on a preset list of diseases and all "public health events of international concern".

Institutions in charge of health security no longer rely solely on traditional disease reporting mechanisms such as mandatory notification of diseases. While these systems can ensure appropriate public health response to identified risks, they cannot recognise the emergence of new threats such as SARS, human cases of avian influenza, or potential deliberate outbreaks. In order to overcome the limitations of traditional surveillance for the detection of previously unknown threats, new approaches have been developed, including the monitoring of syndromes, death rates, health services admissions, or drug prescriptions [11]. These new approaches contribute to enhance the performance of traditional surveillance systems.

Meanwhile, the media and other informal sources of information are increasingly recognised as valuable sources of public health alerts. Epidemic intelligence provides a conceptual framework into which countries may complete their public health surveillance system to meet new challenges [13]. This approach represents a new paradigm aiming at complementing traditional surveillance systems.

The ECDC has in its founding regulation the task to identify and assess emerging threats to human health from communicable diseases. In order to fulfil its mandate, ECDC has developed methods of monitoring potential public health threats from a European perspective [20], under the principle of subsidiarity and building on the experience acquired by the health threat unit of the European Commission and WHO.

7.6 ECDC and Epidemic Intelligence

Since its foundation, the ECDC has developed a structure that combines the evolving methods to identify previously unknown or emerging health threats with traditional routine surveillance systems that include European-wide surveillance networks.

The epidemic intelligence function is one of the fundamental activities at ECDC. The objective is to produce timely and verified intelligence on events of public health interest to be acted upon by public health authorities or medical professionals.

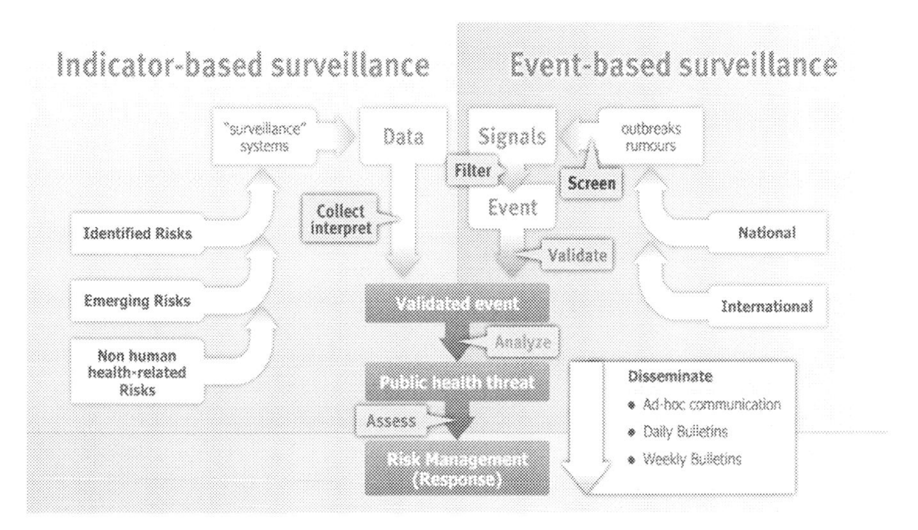

Fig. 7.1 ECDC threat detection framework

The process of epidemic intelligence implies, among other things, the screening of unstructured information (including web, official authorities and media reports). Filtering the relevant events and validating among these unverified information, is part of the process. Epidemic intelligence needs to be understood both as a linear and as a repetitive process. At each repetition the level of information available will change and a new assessment may be needed.

The epidemic intelligence process includes two components: Indicator-based surveillance (IBS) and Event-based surveillance (EBS) [20]. Both components' purpose is to identify public health events. While IBS deals with data that have been previously validated, EBS focuses on media articles, rumours, and other unverified information, that therefore requires validation. The graph in Fig. 7.1 shows the process described, from the IBS/EBS perspective.

When the ECDC became operational in 2005, it began to "gather and analyse data and information on emerging public health threats" (Article 9 of the Founding Regulations of the Centre). According to Article 2(e), health threat "shall mean a condition, agent or incident which may cause, directly or indirectly, ill health". The Founding Regulations further state that ECDC's mission is to "identify, assess and communicate current and emerging threats to human health from communicable diseases" (Article 3(1)). Article 8 states that the ECDC shall "assist the Commission by operating the early warning and response system" and "analyse the content of messages received by it".

The epidemic intelligence process considers emerging threats that are either directly reported to the ECDC through member state notifications on the Early Warning and Response System (EWRS) according to defined criteria [7] or found through active screening of various sources, including national epidemiological bulletins, and international networks such as the Program for Monitoring Emerging Diseases (ProMED-mail), the Global Public Health Intelligence Network (GPHIN), media, and various additional sources, both formal and informal.

The EWRS is the main source of confirmed threats in the EU [9]. It is a dedicated restricted network within the EU for alerts and response, with a legal basis that divides the system into three operational components: an early warning and response system for reporting of specified threats to the public; the exchange of information between accredited structures and authorities of the member states relevant to public health; and specific networks on diseases selected for epidemiological surveillance in the EU member states. The system is hosted and maintained by the ECDC. The EWRS objective is to ensure a rapid and effective response by the EU to events (including emergencies) related to communicable diseases. Competent public health authorities of the member states have to communicate to the network any threat matching a set of defined criteria, by posting a new message. New messages are then followed by comments on the same threat, forming threads of messages. EWRS criteria are the following:

- Outbreaks of communicable diseases extending to more than one Member State of the Community.
- Spatial or temporal clustering of cases of a disease of a similar type if pathogenic agents are a possible cause and there is a risk of propagation between Member States within the Community.
- Spatial or temporal clustering of cases of disease of a similar type outside the Community if pathogenic agents are a possible cause and there is a risk of propagation to the Community.
- The appearance or resurgence of a communicable disease or an infectious agent which may require timely coordinated Community action to contain it.
- Any IHR notification has to be reported also through EWRS.
- Any event related to communicable diseases with a potential EU dimension necessitating contact tracing to identify infected persons or persons potentially in danger may involve the exchange of sensitive personal data of confirmed or suspected cases between concerned Member States.

From January 2005 until the end of 2010, 1,023 new message threads were posted in the EWRS, of which 982 were related to disease threats. In 2010, the number of message threads was similar to previous years excluding the ones related to influenza (Fig. 7.2).

The number of comments – 1,911 – posted as reply to messages in 2010 was also similar to other years, excluding the year 2009, when messages and comments were significantly higher due to the influenza H1N1 pandemic (Fig. 7.3).

An analysis of a 276-week series of new threats, posted in EWRS between 2004 and 2009, shows a positive trend of EWRS use by the member states over the 6-year period. Two outlying data sets emerge: a cluster of events in 2006 attributable to avian influenza (H5N1) and an increase attributable to the H1N1 pandemic in 2009. The average number of new message threads posted per week during the H1N1 pandemic 2009 was 19.16 versus 1.92 during the preceding 5 years, indicating an unprecedented ten-fold increase in reporting during the pandemic period (Fig. 7.4).

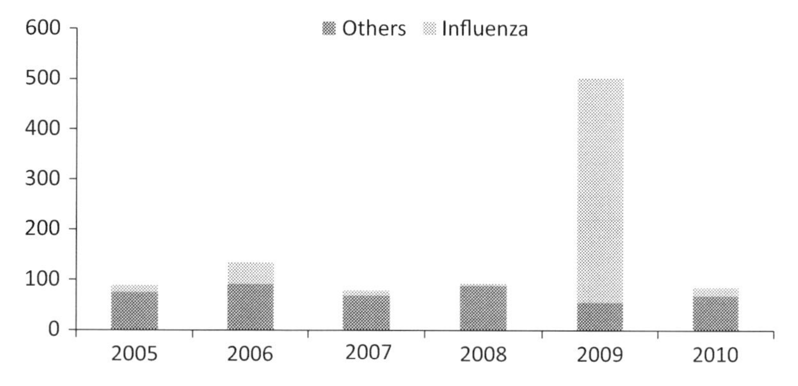

Fig. 7.2 EWRS – Distribution of message threads related to influenza and other pathogens by year of posting

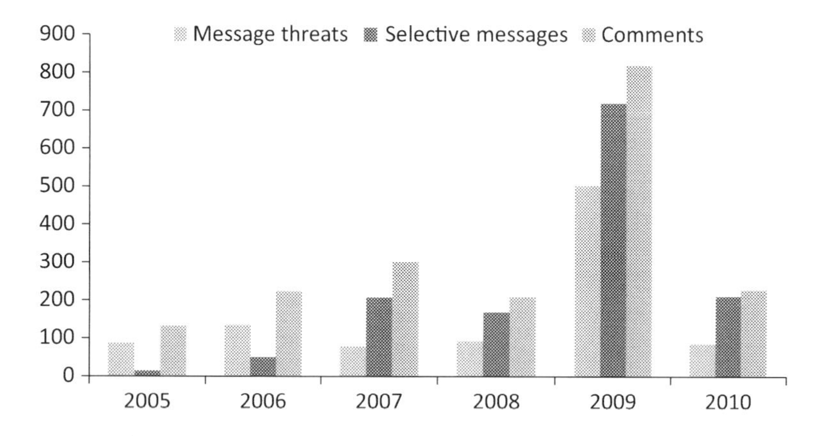

Fig. 7.3 Distribution of EWRS messages by year of posting

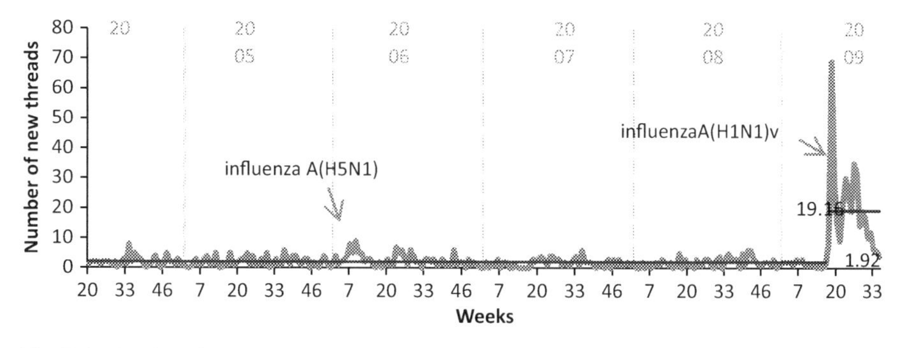

Fig. 7.4 Number of new message threads posted per week in EWRS from week 20/2004 to week 35/2009

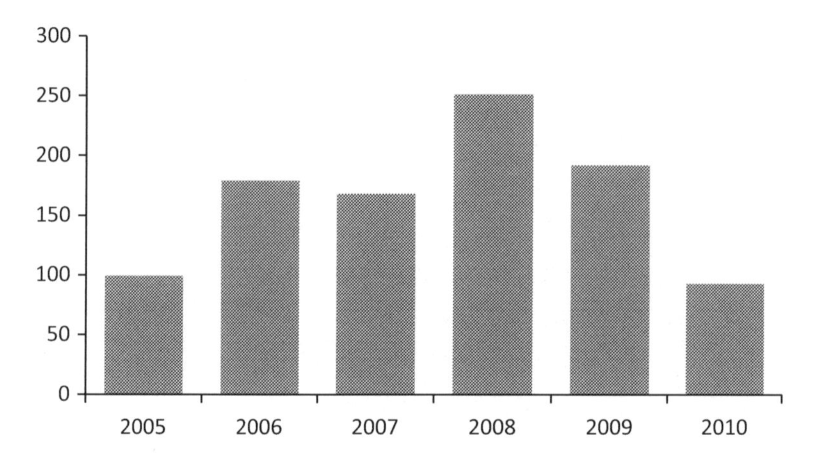

Fig. 7.5 Number of monitored threats by ECDC event-based epidemic intelligence, 2005–2010

The EWRS platform is increasingly used by the EU member states to share information on communicable disease events and facilitate the cross-border coordination of public health measures.

Complementarily, since June 2005, the event-based monitoring of ECDC has recorded about 900 threats, ranging yearly between 93 in 2010 and 251 in 2008 (Fig. 7.5).

Disease-specific surveillance networks, EWRS or information sent to the ECDC by the EU member states or WHO are all considered confidential sources with restricted access. Public sources, on the contrary, are sources accessible on the internet. The main source of new threats is the European Legionnaires' Disease Surveillance Network (ELDSNet). It accounts for nearly a third of newly monitored threats, while EWRS constitutes one fifth of threats monitored by ECDC. The proportion of newly monitored threats originating from confidential sources ranged from 70 to 80% between 2006 and 2010 (Table 7.3).

Some examples of recent threats monitored by ECDC can help understand the added value of a European focus of epidemic intelligence in identifying clustering of cases, assessing their importance to public health, and supporting a multi-country response.

7.6.1 Dengue in Croatia and France

On 13 September 2010, the French Ministry of Health reported the first autochthonous case of dengue fever in metropolitan France. The case was detected through the enhanced routine surveillance system in place from May to October 2010 in areas infested by *Aedes albopictus* in South Eastern France [17]. The information

Table 7.3 Sources of information for newly opened threats at ECDC, by year (EU countries and countries of the European Economic Area)

	Percentage of new threats monitored per year						
Source	2005	2006	2007	2008	2009	2010	Total
Confidential sources							
EPIS for food and water borne diseases						2	0
EWGLI/ELDSNET	2	18	28	34	49	30	29
EWRS	23	32	30	32	24	19	28
WHO	17	9	4	1	2	6	5
Information from member states	1	3	1	3	1	5	2
European disease surveillance networks	9	7	6	2	3	2	4
Other confidential sources		1	3	4	2	11	3
Total percentage	**53**	**70**	**71**	**77**	**80**	**76**	**72**
Public sources							
PROMED	36	9	14	4	3	1	10
MedISYS	2	3			4		2
GPHIN	4	12	3		2		4
Eurosurveillance	0	1	1				0
Public reports available on the Internet	5	6	8	7	5	8	7
Other public sources			2	11	6	14	6
Total percentage	**47**	**30**	**29**	**23**	**20**	**24**	**27**
Total number of threats	**99**	**163**	**142**	**228**	**174**	**83**	**889**

was made available on the public website of the Ministry of Health and through the EWRS on the same day.

The case, residing in Nice (district of Alpes Maritimes) developed symptoms on 23 August 2010 and fully recovered after hospitalisation. Laboratory tests performed in early September confirmed the infection. The case had no history of recent international travel and no blood transfusion.

A second case from the same neighbourhood, presenting onset of symptoms at the beginning of September, was laboratory confirmed on 17 September 2010. These two autochthonous cases of dengue fever were clustered in space and time suggesting an on-going local transmission of dengue. In response to this event, the French authorities have strengthened entomological surveillance in the infested regions and vector control activities in the areas where the cases were reported. Active case finding was implemented in the neighbourhood where cases resided. Communication campaigns for the general public and health professionals also took place [14].

On 30 September 2010, the German health authorities notified through EWRS a laboratory confirmed case of dengue fever in a German citizen returning from Croatia. The patient spent 2 weeks in the beginning of August in Podobuce/Orebić on the Pelješac peninsula, 60 km northwest from Dubrovnik, in the southern part of the country. Considering the onset of symptoms and the incubation period of the disease, the patient was most likely infected during his stay in Croatia [22]. The national health authorities of Croatia took adequate control measures, including raising awareness among health professionals, strengthening human and vector surveillance, implementation of control measures, and communication of personal protective measures to the public. On 22 October 2010 one more case with febrile illness was identified through active case finding in the same village where the infected tourist resided. In addition, 9 of 14 blood samples of healthy individuals living in close proximity suggested recent infection with dengue virus. Further evidence of autochthonous transmission was suggested following a sero-prevalence survey using a random sample of the population living in the area. Five per cent of tested individuals had laboratory indication of recent infection [8, 10].

On 15 September 2010, the ECDC shared a threat assessment for the EU conducted in collaboration with national and disease specific experts of EU member states through the EWRS. The conclusion was that the detection of two autochthonous cases of dengue fever in France and the first autochthonous case in Croatia were significant public health events, but not unexpected. The described events have been the first locally acquired dengue cases reported in continental Europe since 1927–1928, when large dengue outbreaks occurred in Greece. All cases in 2010 occurred in areas known to be infested by *Aedes albopictus* mosquitoes. Previous events, including the chikungunya outbreak in Italy in 2007 [1], the occurrence of vector-borne diseases around airports and other ports of entry, and a previous risk assessment on dengue introduction in the EU [15] indicate that autochthonous transmission of dengue in continental Europe is possible, as confirmed by these events. At the end of the period of mosquito activity, usually in October/November, the risk of establishment of sustained transmission of dengue in south-eastern France and in southern Croatia and further spread in Europe during 2010 appeared very limited. These two events highlighted the need to further strengthen vector monitoring, active surveillance for imported and autochthonous human cases, awareness of health care providers, and laboratory capacities, in countries where *Aedes albopictus* is present, and increase the effectiveness of rapid exchange of information among countries to identify threats and support the response.

7.6.2 Anthrax in Injecting Drug Users

In December 2009, two fatal cases of anthrax in injecting drug users, who had developed symptoms in the first week of December, were reported from Glasgow, Scotland. The initial cluster of five cases in Scotland increased to 47 cases with 16 fatalities until the outbreak was declared over.

In January 2010, one fatal case of anthrax in an injecting drug user was reported from Germany. Even though the strains identified in Germany and Scotland were indistinguishable, no link to Scotland could be established. Two further cases were subsequently identified in Germany. On 5 February 2010, cases started to be reported also in England, the first case coming from the London area. Since the beginning of the outbreak in December 2009, 55 cases of anthrax in injecting drug users have been reported (Scotland 47, England 5, Germany 3), 21 of them fatal (Scotland 16, England 4, Germany 1), resulting in a case fatality rate of 38 %. The last case was reported from Kent, United Kingdom, on 3 November 2010. On 23 December 2010, the outbreak was officially declared over.

In Scotland and England, information was sent out to hospitals, general practitioners, emergency departments, microbiologists and drug services, in order to raise awareness and to request that cases of severe soft tissue infection or sepsis affecting injecting drug users be reported to their local public health authority. Samples of heroin were tested in Scotland in order to identify a possible contaminated batch, but did not yield any positive results. Considering the complex international distribution chain of heroin and the laboratory confirmed link between strains of *Bacillus anthracis* in Scotland and Germany, the exposure to a contaminated batch of heroin distributed in several EU member states seemed probable. However, the source could not be identified and additional cases occurred over the course of the year from the three initially affected areas. Even though skin and soft tissue infections in injecting drug users are common, anthrax as the cause of such infection, especially when fatal, is rare, and very few cases have been described so far [16, 19].

Immediately after the first notifications through EWRS, the ECDC and the European Monitoring Centre for Drugs and Drug Addiction (EMCDDA) issued a joint threat assessment and alerted their networks to gather additional information and to strengthen surveillance to detect possible additional cases in Europe. The threat assessment was updated after the reports about additional cases from England, which suggested a potentially wider spread of the possible source. The European law enforcement agency EUROPOL was also informed and provided support to their law enforcement network in EU member states in attempts to identify a possible deliberate source of contamination.

7.7 Concluding Remarks

Even though information technology and open source intelligence plays an important role in the surveillance activities of the ECDC, the human factor is essential. The use of tools in assisting automated filtering of the vast amount of information available is not yet developed enough to replace expert validation of the information. The production of threat assessments of importance to public health authorities are of little help without properly understanding the context and the consequences of possible measures that can be implemented. Human expertise still makes the difference in making sense of raw information.

The added value of the ECDC in the detection and control of communicable disease threats has not only been proven by the number of threat assessments requested and used for public health decisions, the involvement in support missions for outbreaks and the number of expert meetings organised, but also by the rapid distribution of relevant information through weekly bulletins and postings on the ECDC website and by the contribution to methodological developments in public health security.

References and Further Reading

1. Angelini R et al (2007) An outbreak of chikungunya fever in the province of Ravenna, Italy. Euro Surveill 12(36):pii=3260
2. Coignard B (2001) Bioterrorism preparedness and response in European public health institutes. Euro Surveill 6(11):pii=383
3. COM (2003) Commission of the European Communities. Communication from the Commission to the Council and the European Parliament on cooperation in the European Union on preparedness and response to biological and chemical agent attacks. Brussels, 2 June 2003, COM (2003) 320 final. http://www.sussex.ac.uk/Units/spru/hsp/documents/2003-0602%20Health%20Security.pdf
4. COM (2011) Commission of the European Communities. Commission proposal for a decision of the European Parliament and of the Council on serious cross-border threats to health. Brussels, 8 December 2011, COM (2011) 866 final. http://ec.europa.eu/health/preparedness_response/docs/hsi_proposal_en.pdf
5. Decisions 2000/96 EC, 2003/534 EC and 2119/98 EC
6. EU emergency and crisis co-ordination arrangements. http://www.consilium.europa.eu/uedocs/cmsUpload/WEB15106.pdf
7. EC decision 2000/57/EC and its amendment, decision 2008/351/EC
8. Gjenero-Margan I AB et al. (2011) Autochthonous dengue fever in Croatia, August-September 2010. Euro Surveill 16(9):pii=19805
9. Guglielmetti P et al (2006) The early warning and response system for communicable diseases in the EU: an overview from 1999 to 2005. Euro Surveill 11(12):215–220
10. Health, C.N.I.o.P. (2010) Dengue in Croatia. Epidemiological Bulletin, October 2010
11. Heymann DL, Rodier G (2001) Hot spots in a wired world: WHO surveillance of emerging and re-emerging infectious diseases. Lancet Infect Dis 1(5):345–353
12. HSC, Strategic work plan 2008–2010. http://ec.europa.eu/health/ph_threats/Bioterrorisme/docs/keydo_bio_05_en.pdf
13. Kaiser R, Coulombier D (2006) Different approaches to gathering epidemic intelligence in Europe. Euro Surveill 11(4):E060427.1
14. La Ruche G et al (2010) First two autochthonous dengue virus infections in metropolitan France, September 2010. Euro Surveill 15(39):19676
15. La Ruche G et al (2010) Surveillance par les laboratoires des cas de dengue et de chikungunya importés en France métropolitaine 2008–2009. [Laboratory surveillance of dengue and chikungunya cases imported in metropolitan France 2008–2009]. Bull Epidemiol Hebd 31–32:325–329
16. McGuigan CC et al (2002) Lethal outbreak of infection with Clostridium novyi type A and other spore-forming organisms in Scottish injecting drug users. J Med Microbiol 51(11):971–977
17. Ministre du travail, d.l.e.e.d.l.s.F (2010) Premier cas autochtone isolé de dengue en France métropolitaine. http://www.sante.gouv.fr/premier-cas-autochtone-isole-de-dengue-en-france-metropolitaine.html
18. Monitoring and Information Centre (MIC). http://ec.europa.eu/echo/civil_protection/civil/prote/mic.htm
19. Murray-Lillibridge K et al (2006) Epidemiological findings and medical, legal, and public health challenges of an investigation of severe soft tissue infections and deaths among injecting drug users, Ireland, 2000. Epidemiol Infect 134(4):894–901

20. Paquet C et al (2006) Epidemic intelligence: a new framework for strengthening disease surveillance in Europe. Euro Surveill 11(12):pii=665
21. Regulation (EC) No 851/2004 of the European Parliament and of the Council
22. Schmidt-Chanasit J et al (2010) Dengue virus infection in a traveller returning from Croatia to Germany. Euro Surveill 15(40)
23. Tegnell A et al (2003) The European Commission's taskforce on bioterrorism. EID 9(10):1330–1332
24. Treaty on the functioning of the European Union. http://eur-lex.europa.eu/LexUriServ/LexUriServ.do?uri=OJ:C:2008:115:0047:0199:EN:PDF

Chapter 8
Case Study – Bulgaria

Raynichka Mihaylova-Garnizova and Kamen Plochev

Abstract The aim of this paper is to map the current situation in Bulgaria's public healthcare system with regard to bioterrorism response. It explores the main public health threats and focuses specifically on the changing perception of bioterrorism as a potential threat to the country. Furthermore, it explains how this perception is reflected in the existing legal framework and administrative structures. The paper makes the case for the further development of an integrated, flexible and sustainable national management system to respond effectively to emergencies and presents the major challenges for the country in this field. It makes a comparison between military and civilian agencies in their preparedness to respond to naturally occurring emergencies and threats of biological attack. This review points out the higher but still limited capacity of the military medical facilities in Bulgaria. The overall evaluation underlines the need for further strengthening of the relationship between military and civil capabilities and between public healthcare and security and law enforcement structures. As a result the authors make the case for stronger cooperation between military and civil medical facilities as well as for inter-institutional and interdisciplinary dialogue on the expert and political level on biopreparedness in Bulgaria.

8.1 Introduction

The aim of this contribution is to map the current situation in Bulgaria's public healthcare system with regard to bioterrorism response.

In Bulgaria public health and biopreparedness are still regarded as two independent public policies. Public health, including control of infectious diseases and the

R. Mihaylova-Garnizova (✉) • K. Plochev
Department of Infectious Diseases, Military Medical Academy,
Clinic of Infectious Diseases, Sofia, Bulgaria
e-mail: doctor.mihaylova@gmail.com

I. Hunger et al. (eds.), *Biopreparedness and Public Health: Exploring Synergies*,
NATO Science for Peace and Security Series A: Chemistry and Biology,
DOI 10.1007/978-94-007-5273-3_8, © Springer Science+Business Media Dordrecht 2013

counter of epidemics, is a priority of the Ministry of Health while preparation for response to bioterrorism is almost entirely within the scope of the activities of the Ministry of Defence. Moreover, until recently the efforts of the military experts were focused completely on the problems of biodefence in the event of an attack with biological weapons and the basic protection of the army. On one hand, the prioritization of the protection of the civilian population from bioterrorism on the global scene in general, and the emergence of new epidemics of infectious diseases, on the other hand, naturally impose the need for coherence and cooperation of efforts of different institutions in Bulgaria for responding to bioterrorism.

Furthermore, in the beginning, a covert biological attack cannot be distinguished straightforwardly from a naturally occurring epidemic, in which case the response will be handled by the existing public health structures.

The overall evaluation is that Bulgaria has no experience in countering bioterrorism.

8.2 Current Public Health Threats and Perceptions

The main public health threats concerning infectious diseases in Bulgaria are defined in the Health Act and its additional regulations. About 60 diseases are indicated in the official list of infectious and parasitic diseases, which are subject to mandatory registration, notification and reporting (Table 8.1). However, not all of the items in the list are subject to regular monitoring. Regular updates are given for 50% of the infectious diseases.

The data for morbidity of the most important communicable diseases for the country is published in the weekly epidemiological bulletin (Table 8.2), published by the National Centre for Infectious and Parasitic Diseases.

Contrary to the existing infectious diseases list, Bulgarian authorities do not have an established official list of potential agents for bioterrorism. In a recent publication we have proposed a list of bio-agents (Table 8.3) which represent a potential threat for Bulgarian citizens in case of bioterrorism, taking into account the following criteria [5]:

- Bulgaria's geographical position;
- The immunization calendar of the country; and
- The implementation of commitments to peacekeeping and other missions.

This lack of official position on the threat of biological agents needs to be further clarified. Until very recently according to the Bulgarian authorities there was no risk of terrorism in the country, including risk of bioterrorism. This attitude is changing and the new position of the government is that Bulgaria faces the risks and threats common to the Euro-Atlantic area which include terrorism and weapons of mass destruction.

The new National Security Strategy of the Republic of Bulgaria (NSS), adopted by the National Assembly on 25 February 2011, states that "risks and threats (including bioterrorism) to the security of the Republic of Bulgaria and its citizens largely coincide or are similar to those that threaten other EU countries and NATO" [4].

Table 8.1 Official list of infectious and parasitic diseases

1. Amebiasis
2. Anthrax
3. Ascariasis
4. Bacterial meningitis and meningo-encephalitis:
4.1. With specified etiology
4.1.1. Pneumococcal
4.1.2. Streptococcal
4.1.3. Haemophilus influenzae
4.1.4. Other bacteria
4.2. With unspecified etiology
5. Botulism
6. Brucellosis
7. Rabies
8. Creutzfeldt-Jakob disease
9. Smallpox
10. Chickenpox
11. Viral meningitis and meningo-encephalitis
12. Viral haemorrhagic fevers:
12.1. Ebola and Marburg fever
12.2. Lassa fever
12.3. Congo-Crimean haemorrhagic fever
12.4. Haemorrhagic fever with renal syndrome
13. Viral hepatitis:
13.1. Acute viral hepatitis types A, B, C, D, unidentified
13.2. Chronic viral hepatitis type B, C, D
14. Gastroenteritis, enterocolitis
15. Gonococcal infection
16. Influenza and acute respiratory infections (ARI)
17. Shigellosis
18. Diphtheria
19. Mumps
20. Echinococcosis
21. Yellow fever
22. Yersiniosis
23. Campylobacteriosis
24. Pertussis
25. Enterohaemorrhagic *E. coli* infection
26. Typhoid fever
27. Cryptosporidiosis
28. Q fever
29. Lyme borreliosis
30. Leishmaniosis, visceral
31. Lambliosis
32. Legionellosis
33. Leptospirosis
34. Listeriosis
35. Malaria

(continued)

Table 8.1 (continued)

36. Marseilles fever (Mediterranean spotted fever (MSF))
37. Meningococcal infection (meningo-coccal meningitis and sepsis)
38. Measles
39. Ornithosis
40. Spotted fever
41. Poliomyelitis
41.1. Acute Flaccid Paralysis
42. Rubella
42.1. Congenital rubella
43. Salmonellosis
44. Syndrome of acquired immune deficiency (AIDS) and HIV infection
45. Syphilis
46. Scarlet fever
47. Streptococcus pneumoniae, invasive infection
48. Severe acute respiratory syndrome (SARS)
49. Tapeworm infection (*Taenia solium*, *Taenia saginata*, *Hymenolepis nana*, and *Diphyllobothrium latum*)
50. Tetanus
51. Toxoplasmosis
52. Trichinosis
53. Tuberculosis
54. Tularaemia
55. Haemophilus influenzae type B invasive infection
56. Chlamydia trachomatis, genital infection
57. Cholera
58. Plague

Table 8.2 Epidemiological bulletin list

Anthrax	Lyme borreliosis
Bacterial meningitis and meningo-encephalitis	Legionellosis
Botulism	Leptospirosis
Brucellosis	Listeriosis
Chickenpox	Marseilles fever (Mediterranean spotted fever (MSF))
Crimean-Congo haemorrhagic fever	Meningococcal infection (meningo-coccal meningitis and sepsis)
Viral meningitis and meningo-encephalitis	Ornithosis
Gastroenteritis, enterocolitis	Acute viral hepatitis types A, B, C, D
Congenital rubella	Rubella
Shigellosis	Salmonellosis
Mumps	Scarlet fever
Pertussis	Tetanus
Yersiniosis	Tularaemia
Campylobacteriosis	Haemorrhagic fever with renal syndrome
E. coli enterocolitis	Chronic viral hepatitis type B, C, D
Typhoid fever	

Table 8.3 Proposed list of bio-agents which represent a potential threat for Bulgarian citizens in case of bioterrorism

Bacterial agents	Viral agents	Biological toxins
B. anthracis	SARS CoV	Botulinum toxin
Brucella spp.	H5N1	Ricin
B. mallei	H1N1	SEB
B. pseudomallei	Orthopox virus	T-2 mycotoxins
Y. pestis	Venezuelan equine encephalitis virus	
F. tularensis	Haemorrhagic fever viruses	
V. cholera		
Rickettsia	*C. burnetii*	

The strategy gives special attention to asymmetric threats, especially international terrorism and proliferation of weapons of mass destruction (WMD) and their impact on security in a global and regional context. The document underlines the increasing possibilities of the use of radioactive materials, toxic substances and biological agents, as well as access to information databases and technology for the combat of terrorism.

Particular attention is paid to a number of issues:

- Surveillance of communicable diseases;
- Country protection from importation and distribution of infections;
- Outbreak reduction;
- Terrorist use of biological agents;
- High immunization coverage of the population;
- Rapid response organisations in situations threatening public health;
- Specific actions taken to prevent widespread disease among vulnerable and marginalized populations.

The new approach indicates the importance of building an integrated, flexible and sustainable national management system to respond effectively to crises. In order to reach an effective crisis management level, it is necessary to develop integrated military and civilian capabilities for action in the country and the EU.

This new orientation in the strategic thinking has not been further developed into procedures and other types of documents, including officially recognized bio-threat agents.

8.3 Response to Emergencies

8.3.1 Legal Framework

The perception of risk reflected in the new National Security Strategy and the necessity of integrated military and civilian capabilities fully correspond to the existing legal framework. Firstly, it should be pointed out that the current legal framework reflects the changes that have occurred in Bulgaria in the past few years. Secondly, the framework has been fully revised in light of Bulgaria's membership in NATO and the European Union. As a result, Bulgarian authorities have aimed at achieving full alignment with internationally acknowledged crisis management systems. Even though an overall look at the existing framework, reveals a strong foundation for Bulgaria's anti-terrorism and WMD defence policies, a deeper observation shows lack of a strategy explicitly addressing the threat and response to bioterrorism [1].

The key acts and plans in Bulgaria on these topics are listed below for information. However, their full description and evaluation is beyond the scope and focus of this paper.

- The Defence and Armed Forces Act
- Ministry of Interior Act
- Healthcare Act
- National Security Strategy of The Republic of Bulgaria
- Law on Disaster Protection
- The Terrorism Management Plan
- National programme for strengthening the capacity of Bulgaria for the prevention of importation of infectious diseases and reaction in events, presenting danger for public health for 2008–2010

8.3.2 Overall Coordination of Managing Bodies

The following governmental bodies are engaged in emergency response and preparedness, including in the case of a bioterrorist threat (Fig. 8.1):

- The Ministry of Health;
- The Ministry of Defence;
- The Ministry of Interior;
- The Ministry of Agriculture and Food;
- State Agency for National Security;
- State Agency "State Reserve and War-time Stock";
- State Agency "Civil Protection" of the Ministry of Interior.

The Council of Ministers (CM) has the overall responsibility for the design and the implementation of the disaster prevention policy. It adopts the national disaster relief plan and annual strategies for its implementation. The Council establishes the Inter-Ministerial Commission for Recovery and Assistance (ICRA) with representation from the Ministry of Finance (MF), Economics, Energy and Tourism (MEET), Defence (MD), Transport, Information Technologies and Communication (MTITC), Agriculture and Food (MAF), and Health (MH). The Council of Ministers delegates to the Minister of Interior (MI) the responsibility to establish and manage the activities of the Integrated Rescue System (IRS). The IRS organizes,

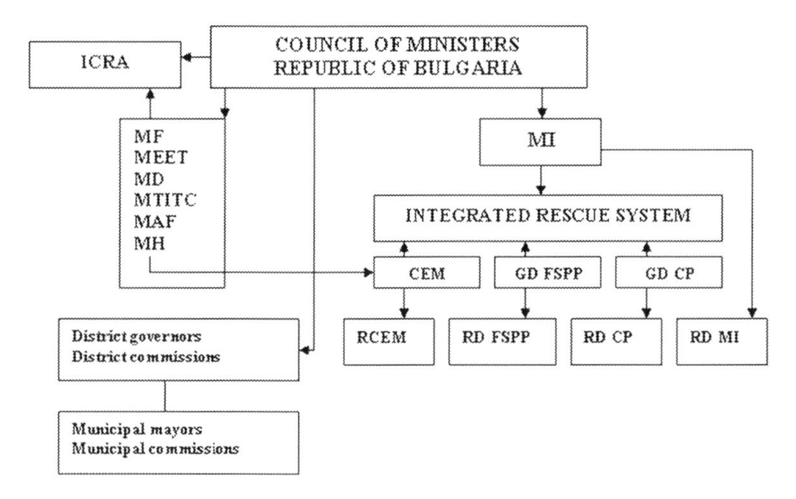

CEM	Centres for Emergency Medicine
GDCP	General Direction "Civil Protection"
GDFSPP	General Direction "General Fire Safety and Protection of Population"
ICRA	Inter-Ministerial Commission for Recovery and Assistance
MAF	Ministry of Agriculture and Food
MD	Ministry of Defence
MEET	Ministry of Economics, Energy and Tourism
MF	Ministry of Finance
MH	Ministry of Health
MI	Minister of Interior
MTITC	Ministry of Transport, Information Technologies and Communication
RCEM	Regional Centres for Emergency Medicine
RDCP	Regional Direction "Civil Protection"
RDFSPP	Regional Direction "General Fire Safety and Protection of Population"
RDMI	Regional Directions of the Ministry of Interior

Fig. 8.1 Interaction of managing bodies

coordinates and manages the activities of the bodies and structures taking part in disaster relief.

The IRS includes the General Direction "Civil Protection" (GDCP), the General Direction "General Fire Safety and Protection of Population" (GDFSPP) and the regional directions of the Ministry of Interior, as well as the Centres for Emergency Medicine (CEM) and its regional divisions of the Ministry of Health. The main components of the IRS are present in all districts and municipalities throughout the country. In case of a disaster, the chief of operations manages and coordinates the activities of territorial units of IRS on the scene. This position is held by the chief of the territorial unit of the GDFSPP. In the case of epidemics, the activities on the scene are managed by the director of the Regional Health Inspection.

In the following sections, we will have a detailed look at the key bodies involved in emergency response.

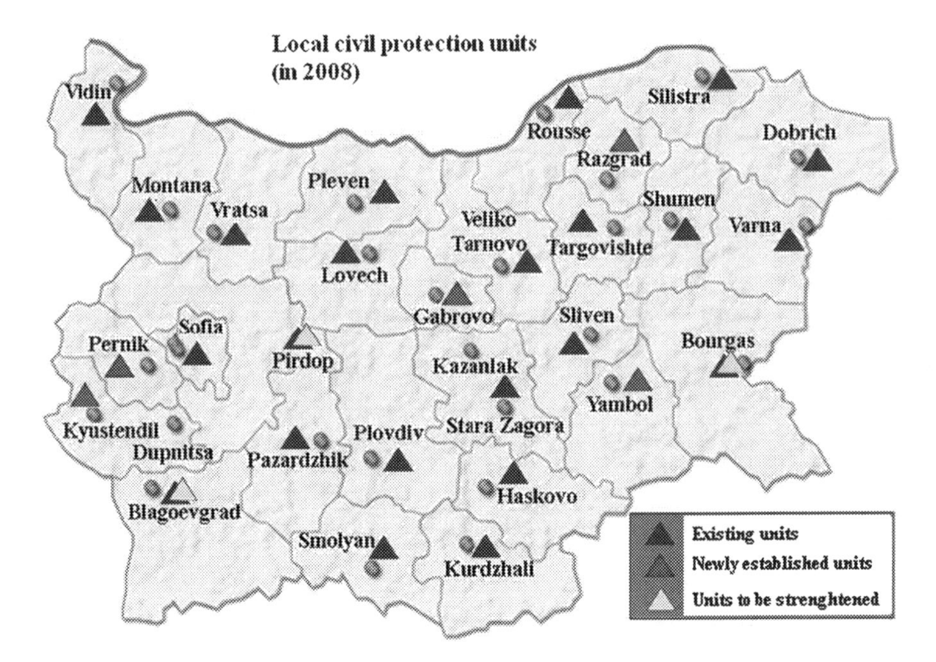

Fig. 8.2 Local civil protection assets

8.3.3 General Direction "Civil Protection"

General Direction "Civil Protection" (GDCP), part of the Ministry of Interior, currently performs a number of tasks related to disaster relief. Firstly, the body warns and signals of the threat of a disaster which also includes the case of state of war (Fig. 8.2). Secondly, it performs search and rescue operations during disasters, including emergency works. In case of incidents and emergencies related to harmful materials and substances, the General Direction is in charge of radiation, chemical and biological protection. In terms of actions for prevention, GDCP organizes education activities and trainings of the population to react during disasters as well as the implementation of protective measures.

Even though GDCP has substantial functions in emergency prevention and response, it lacks tasks directly involved in the use of bioweapons or naturally developing pandemics. In addition to this drawback in its role, it also lacks medical personnel. For this reason GDCP is working in close coordination with the Centres of Emergency Medicine (CEM).

8.3.4 State Agency "State Reserve and War-Time Stocks"

State Agency "State Reserve and War-Time Stocks" is the specialized body of the Council of Ministers that pursues the state policy in the field of the accumulation, maintenance and use of the country's state reserves and war-time stocks in accordance with the national security's interests. (State Agency "State Reserve and War-Time Stocks") More precisely, it organizes and controls the accumulation, maintenance, updating and accounting of the state reserves and war-time stocks [6].

Its functions include:

- Proposals to the Council of Ministers for approval of the state reserves' nomenclature and norms;
- Reports of its activities to the Council of Ministers and to the Inter-Ministerial Commission for Recovery and Assistance (ICRA) in the matter of the military-industrial complex and mobilization training of the country;
- Participation in the international cooperation, European and Euro-Atlantic integration activities.

In Bulgaria, the main stocks piled into the system of state reserves, for which the State Agency is responsible, are: fuels, chemicals, foods, ferrous and non-ferrous metals, spare parts, timbers and paper, medical provisions, hospital equipment, and tools.

In case of a biological attack these are the available resources of the agency. It has the main equipment in terms of medical provisions except serums and vaccines which are kept at the National Centre of Infectious and Parasitic Diseases.

8.3.5 State Agency for National Security

The State Agency for National Security (SANS) was created in 2007 and it is still in the process of development. The State Agency for National Security is a specialized body for counter-intelligence and security and its chief responsibility is to detect, prevent and neutralize the threats to the Bulgarian national security [7].

In order to fulfil its duties, SANS uses in its work the whole spectrum of counter-intelligence means and resources. The Agency operates against the classic intelligence and non-traditional threats and risks, provides government authorities with information needed for the decision making in the national security sphere. One of its tasks is the gathering of information regarding time, location and media of dissemination of the biological agent.

Moreover, with respect to prevention of terrorism, including bioterrorism, the Agency performs tasks of surveillance, detection, counteraction and prevention of:

- International trade in weapons, products and technologies of dual use, manufacture, storage and proliferation of items of a generally hazardous nature;
- International terrorism and extremism and their financing;
- Protection of facilities or activities of a strategic nature;
- Actions of groups or persons with support of alien services, terrorist or extremist organizations;
- Disruptive actions on communication and information systems;
- Risks and threats related to migration.

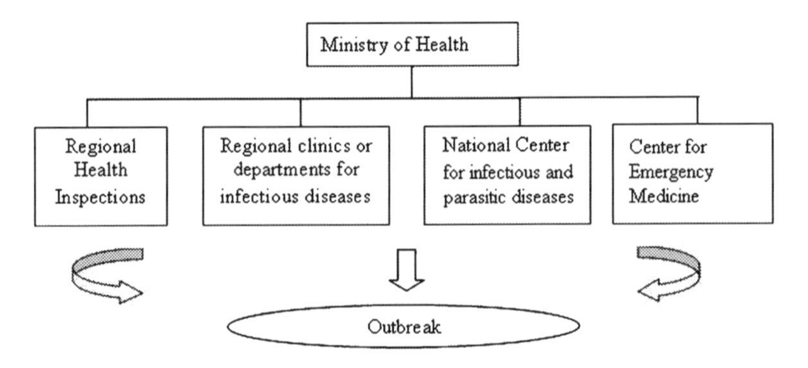

Fig. 8.3 Ministry of Health and its structures

The main concern under discussion about SANS's functions and activities is the order, volume and use of the acquired and analyzed information for the planning to counter a biological attack made by other authorities. This problem stems from the lack of publicity of the reports evaluating the risk of bioterrorism. Therefore, due to the classified nature of the information, further estimates about the activities performed by SANS with respect to biological threats cannot be made.

8.3.6 *Ministry of Health and Its Structures*

The Ministry of Health's main functions encompass two of its strategic goals with respect to emergency response (Fig. 8.3). First of all, it is responsible for surveillance, prevention and protection from infectious diseases. Second, it deals with the organization of the medical response in the case of a biological attack. The structures directly involved in performing these two functions are the National Centre for Infectious and Parasitic Diseases (NCIPD), Regional Health Inspections (RHIs), the Centre for Emergency Medicine and the medical facilities throughout the country (regional clinics or departments for infectious diseases).

The Ministry of Health has issued a plan for public protection in the case of disasters including terrorism, as well as counteraction to an influenza pandemic, but the structures of the Ministry do not have a specific plan for actions in case of biological attack.

8.3.7 *National Centre for Infectious and Parasitic Diseases*

As a result of its efforts in the research and surveillance on infectious diseases, in 2007 the European Centre for Disease Control (ECDC) in Stockholm declared

NCIPD as a leading "national competent body" in the field of infectious and parasitic diseases.

The NCIPD has the status of scientific organization of the Ministry of Health, which aims to develop a scientific basis for the fight against infectious diseases and methods for its implementation. Therefore, the areas of intensive research are: infectious diseases, immune reactivity, epidemiology, laboratory diagnostics, and treatment and prophylaxis of bacterial, viral, and parasitic infections. NCIPD includes all National Reference Laboratories (NRL) in various bacterial, viral and parasitic infections.

The NCIPD, acting in cooperation with the European Centre for Disease Prevention and Control, has developed the capacity for surveillance of the spread of infectious diseases and the modern diagnostic capabilities for Biohazard Level III infections. The reaction to the bird flu pandemic has demonstrated this capacity. The Centre is capable of observing the dissemination of one biological agent, but is not designated to coordinate activities to stop it.

The NCIPD holds the country's reserves of serums and vaccines to be used in cases of biological attack and epidemics. NCIPD has developed a plan for a bio-response; however, access to the documentation is restricted.

8.3.8 Regional Health Inspections

The Regional Health Inspections (RHIs) replaced and merged the functions of the Regional Inspectorate for Protection and Control of Public Health and the Regional Health Centres. The new body started working in January 2011 and it is still in the process of its development.

The RHIs include the regional authorities, performing practical activities concer ning public health, such as the identification of the source of communicable diseases, epidemiological studies and health education activities. Similar to the case with its two predecessors, the Ministry of Health has not delegated tasks to the inspections related to planning its activities in case of a bioterrorist attack.

8.3.9 Civilian Medical Facilities

In addition to the NCIPD and the Regional Health Inspections, the Ministry of Health manages civilian medical facilities which include hospitals, clinics or departments dealing with infectious diseases on the regional, municipal, and district levels.

The civilian medical facilities have the necessary experience to respond to the most common epidemics, but lack the capacity – administrative, personnel and material – to act during a bio-attack.

8.4 Role of the Ministry of Defence and the Military Medical Academy

The state structures having both the capacity and preparedness to act in case of bioterrorism are the Ministry of Defence and the Military Medical Academy (MMA), responsible for the medical treatment of the army [2]. That is why MMA is the only organization able to ensure protection both for the military forces and the civilian population during a bio-attack.

The Military Medical Academy (MMA) was established in 1989, at the Ministry of Defence of the Republic of Bulgaria, as an integrated complex for medical care, education and scientific research with the commitment to develop the military medical science, and to provide training, specialization and qualification of the military medical staff for the purpose of ensuring the fighting strength and combat readiness of the Bulgarian Armed Forces, preservation and recovery of the military servicemen's health. (Military Medical Academy)

Since February 2001, MMA is composed of the following structures for outpatient and hospital care (Fig. 8.4). The Medical Hospitals (MHs) for active treatment are located in Sofia, Varna, Plovdiv, Sliven and Pleven. MMA also includes Centres for Rehabilitation in Hissar, Pomorie and Bankya. In addition, MMA supports the Research Centre for Radiological, Biological and Chemical Protection, the Centre for Military Epidemiology and Hygiene, and Military Medical Units for Emergency Response and its divisions.

Additionally to the above mentioned bodies, MMA operates military medical departments and troops for the army, the air forces and the navy. At the same time, the Central Depot in Lovech holds additional stockpiles in the case of a bio-threat. The MMA develops and regularly updates an action plan for response in case of biological threat which concerns all of MMA's structures.

The Clinic of Infectious Diseases (CID) in Sofia (Fig. 8.5) was reconstructed in 2005 as a result of a military project initiated after the international meetings of experts on biological weapons in Warsaw in January 2003 and Geneva in October 2003. The goal was to build hospital facilities for the reception, isolation and treatment of patients with infectious diseases, and especially for dangerous infections, naturally occurring outbreaks and response to a potential biological attack [3].

The reconstructed clinic fits the modern construction and technology requirements to prevent disease transmission and reduce morbidity of the victims of naturally occurring epidemics and those from biological attack.

The clinic is located in a separate building, which allows protection to prevent the spread of infections in other medical departments of the hospital in Sofia. CID has:

- Capability for isolation and treatment of especially dangerous infections of the bio-safety level 2 and 3;
- Access through a main road and by helicopter;
- Trained medical personnel for bio-attack situations.

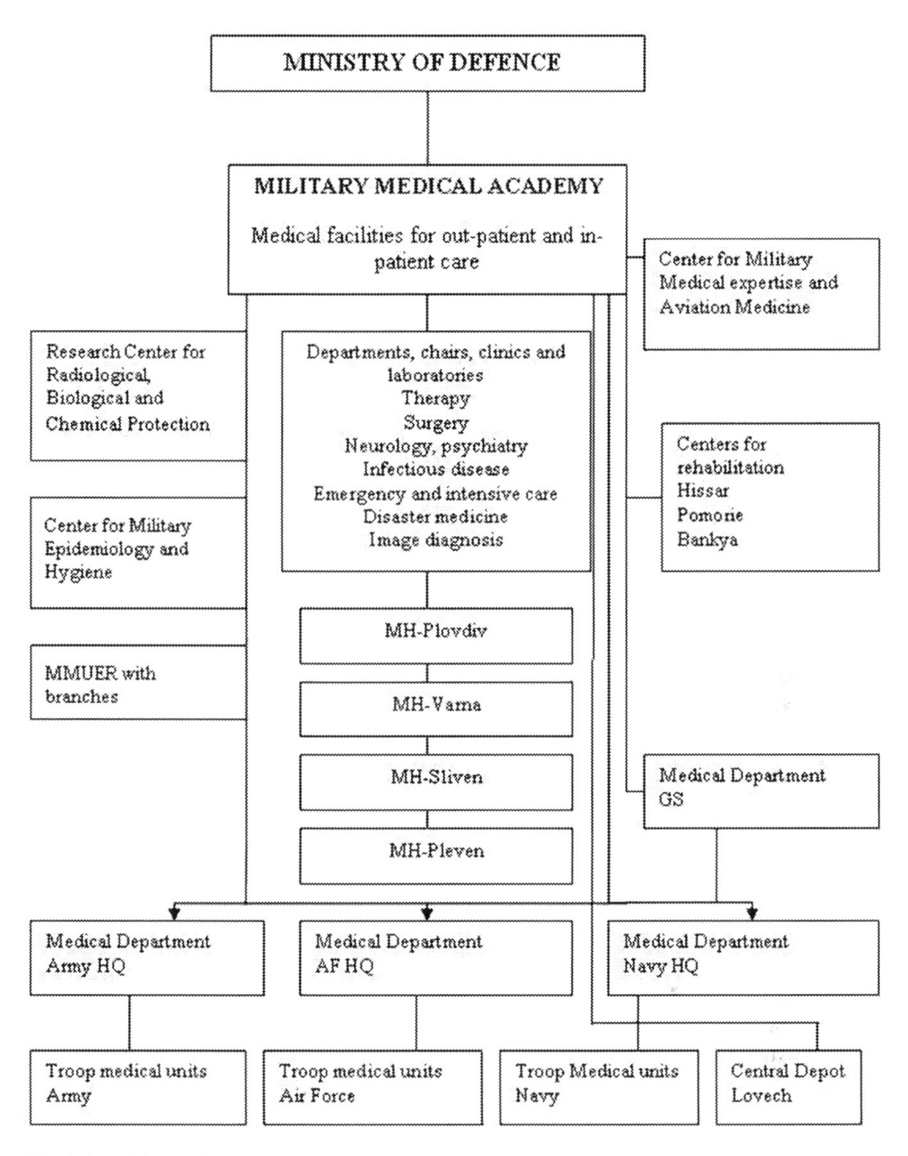

Fig. 8.4 Ministry of Defence and Military Medical Academy

Contrary to the Clinic of Infectious Diseases in Sofia, other military hospitals in the country do not have the same capacity for response to bio-threats. Since other hospitals lack plans, resources and trained personnel, in the case of bio-attack they will be assisted by CID, the Military Medical Unit for Emergency Response, and mobile military hospitals. The latter are intended to be used in these regional military hospitals, which do not have infectious wards.

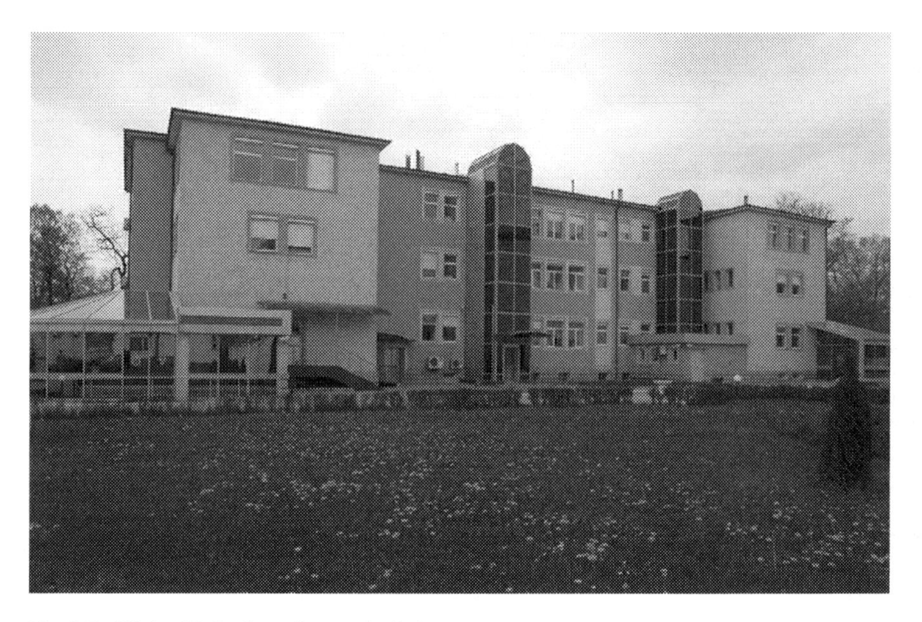

Fig. 8.5 Clinic of infectious diseases in Sofia

8.5 Military-Civilian Partnership

As a general scenario, the military hospitals without infectious wards sign agreements with the civilian hospitals in the same city or region for the transfer of patients. The issue with these agreements is that regardless of the availability of beds they lack the resources for an adequate response to a bio-attack. For this reason the agreements foresee that civilian hospitals will receive support from the medical personnel of MMA.

Both military and civilian hospitals suffer serious shortages of infectious disease professionals which number about 150 medical doctors for the entire country. This is the result of the policies of the Ministry of Health and the National Health Insurance Fund (NHIF) which fail to assure the necessary budget line for infectious diseases.

An issue which has not been subject to public and expert discussions is the interaction between public (civilian and military) and private facilities in case of a bio-attack. This is the case due to the rising number of privately owned hospitals which operate within the network of public healthcare financed by the National Health Insurance Fund even though they do not have any responsibility in naturally occurring epidemics and bio-attacks.

8.6 Conclusion

To sum up, firstly the subject of bioterrorism and preparedness in Bulgaria is fairly new. However, the institutions involved have started developing a strategic approach for this possibility. These efforts are limited by the continuous changes in the legal framework and the implementing structure. The changes are reflected to a lower extent in the organizations responsible for naturally occurring epidemics.

Secondly, in this changing environment the military medical structures hold the highest capacity in emergency response to bio-threats. Here as well, the capacity remains below the necessary level. Regardless of this fact, since the resources in the country for the prevention of bioterrorism are very limited and the health care system is undergoing serious reform, the military medical capacity could be used to protect civilians.

Thirdly, as a result of the limited capability and resources, the need for cooperation is increasing. In some cases this is already the case, while in others the gap has to be addressed even further. The most important of these are the relationship between the public healthcare and preparedness for bioterrorism and the relationship between the public healthcare and security and law enforcement structures. The inter-institutional and interdisciplinary discourse in Bulgaria on the expert and political level is yet to come.

References and Further Reading

1. Disaster Relief Act (2011) Official gazette. 25 January 2011. http://www.lex.bg/bg/laws/ldoc/2135540282. Accessed 30 Apr 2011
2. Military Medical Academy (2011) http://www.vma.bg/indexen.php. Accessed 30 Apr 2011
3. Mihaylova-Garnizova R (2011) Organization of the activities of the medical facilities of the Military Medical Academy in response to a biological attack. PhD thesis, Sofia, MMA
4. National Assembly of the Republic of Bulgaria (2011) National Security Strategy. 25 February 2011. http://www.strategy.bg/FileHandler.ashx?fileId=1419. Accessed 30 Apr 2011
5. Plochev K (2011) Medical activities organization within Bulgarian Army to counter in case of biological weapon usage. DMS thesis, Sofia, MMA
6. State Agency "State Reserve and War-Time Stocks" (2011) http://www.statereserve.bg/dadrvvz/opencms/menu/en/. Accessed 30 Apr 2011
7. State Agency for National Security (2011) http://www.dans.bg/. Accessed 30 Apr 2011

Chapter 9
Case Study – France

Elisande Nexon

Abstract Emerging health risks, weapons of mass destruction, and terrorism – including biological weapons and bioterrorism – are identified in the 2008 White Paper on defence and national security as threats for France and its citizens. Since the beginning of the century, the 2001 anthrax attacks in the USA and subsequent hoaxes as well as the global SARS outbreak and influenza pandemic threats have all contributed to raise public awareness about health emergencies, leading authorities to adapt and improve planning for such events. This chapter focuses on natural and intentional public health threats and on biopreparedness from a French perspective, describing legal and organizational frameworks, plans and guidelines.

9.1 Introduction

The scope of public health threats encompasses epidemics and pandemics, known and (re)-emerging pathogens, accidental releases or contamination, but also malevolence and bioterrorism [8]. As the European Security Strategy identifies threats facing the European Union, the French White Paper on defence and national security (2008) identifies a number of threats and vulnerabilities for France and its citizens. Among these are weapons of mass destruction, terrorism, and emerging health risks, and the issue of the rising number of French citizens living abroad. Other identified vulnerabilities are ballistic and missile threats, major attacks against information systems, new and robust espionage activities, major criminal networks, natural catastrophes, as well as industrial disasters and technological risks. The strategy also integrates four new security parameters: the growing interconnection between

E. Nexon (✉)
Fondation pour la recherche stratégique, Paris, France
e-mail: e.nexon@frstrategie.org

I. Hunger et al. (eds.), *Biopreparedness and Public Health: Exploring Synergies*, NATO Science for Peace and Security Series A: Chemistry and Biology,
DOI 10.1007/978-94-007-5273-3_9, © Springer Science+Business Media Dordrecht 2013

threats and risks resulting from globalization, continuity between domestic and foreign security, the possibility of sudden strategic disruptions, as well as developments impacting military operations.

From a French point of view, surveillance and assessment of public health threats require taking into account metropolitan France, as well as overseas departments and territories spanning three continents. Due to the increasing circulation of goods and people, monitoring of events at the international level is also a requirement, aimed at detecting and characterizing health threats which could affect the French population nationally or abroad. This case study mainly focuses on major threats linked to infectious diseases, be they natural or intentional.

9.2 Infectious Diseases: Trends and Threats

The 2010 annual report of the French National Institute for Public Health Surveillance (InVS) highlights that infectious diseases trends in France include a recurrence of measles, due to inadequate vaccine coverage, and increases in sexually transmitted diseases such as gonococcal infections, as well as a higher incidence of invasive pneumococcal infections. In addition, development of drug resistant strains is a public health challenge. Emerging carbapenem-resistant *Enterobacteriaceae* are for example considered worrisome, even if few cases have been detected in France until now. The 2010 *Bulletin Epidémiologique Hebdomadaire* (BEH) about surveillance assessments of infectious diseases, published by InVS, also underlines the risk of introduction of chikungunya and dengue viruses by travelers arriving or returning from endemic areas, as a potential vector (a mosquito, *Aedes albopictus*) is now present in Southeastern France. In 2008, according to Inserm – CépiDc data, mortality caused by infectious and parasitic diseases represented 2% of the deaths in France.

Regarding potential major health threats, epidemic and pandemic threats remains a great cause for concern, as the dedicated interdepartmental website and national plan show. In 2004, following the SARS outbreak, a new chapter about serious health threats was inserted in the Public Health Code. It is worth noting that the scope of this chapter encompasses all kind of threats, including intentional ones, as bioterrorism is also a concern.

Biopreparedness takes into account agents responsible for anthrax, botulism, plague, smallpox, tularemia, and viral hemorrhagic fevers, all listed in the CDC category A of high-priority agents including organisms that pose a risk for national security. They are among 30 diseases requiring mandatory written reporting, ruled by Article L.3113-1 of the Public Health Code, completed with articles D.3113.6 and D.3113.7 which establish the list. Also, authorities published guidelines and factsheets explaining how to react in the context of a bioterrorist event involving one of these agents or some others.

Except for smallpox, which has been eradicated, these diseases still also represent natural public health threats, even if there are no or few cases. Even if the annual incidence is very low in France, mainly with foodborne cases, the occurrence of unusual and severe cases of botulism provides additional reasons for continuing surveillance [6]. According to 2010 InVS epidemiological data, there are also few cases of tularemia, the reporting of which became mandatory in 2002. Reporting of anthrax cases has been mandatory since 2003, but cases are extremely rare with only one imported case (2003) and three patients infected with cutaneous anthrax (2008) reported in the last decade [5]. Regarding plague, the last cases occurred in 1945. However, this disease is endemic in some areas in Africa and Asia that have close links to France. As for viral hemorrhagic fevers, most cases in metropolitan France are caused by Puumala virus (Hantavirus), responsible for a relatively mild form of hemorrhagic fever with renal symptoms, and yellow fever (Arbovirus) for which vaccination is mandatory to travel to French Guiana. No case of African hemorrhagic fever has been identified in France since the inclusion of these diseases on the mandatory reporting list, however, the risk of importation must not be ignored.

9.3 Serious Public Health Threats and Biopreparedness

9.3.1 Organization at National Level

The General Secretariat for Defence and National Security (SGDSN), reporting to the Prime Minister and working closely with the President of the Republic's office, is responsible for risks and threats assessment, as well as planning and inter-ministerial coordination regarding prevention and response to major threats, including CBRNE terrorist threats and public health threats such as pandemics. According to article L.1141-1 of the Defence Code, each ministry is then responsible for preparation and implementation of incumbent defence measures.

Considering terrorism issues, the CBRNE Strategic Committee was created in 2008, as required in the White Paper. It coordinates the definition of joint orientations and monitors their implementation. Chaired by the Secretary General for Defence and National Security, it convenes representatives from relevant ministries (Ministries of Interior, Health, Defence, Industry, Agriculture, Transports and Budget), and thus aims at ensuring coherence and complementarities. Its role also includes considering how scientific and technological developments can meet operational requirements.

The CBRNE prevention and response plan relies on a number of texts. The 2009 French State Doctrine for the Prevention and Response to CBRNE Terrorism ("Circulaire n°747/SGDN/PSE/PPS, 30 October 2009") defines the framework and identifies ten objectives (Fig. 9.1), each corresponding to a number of specific missions and activities. The interministerial system to address CBRN terrorist threats is specifically described in another document ("Circulaire interministérielle n°007/SGDN/PSE/PPS, 8 October 2009").

Organization, planning, training	1. Organization of the action of State administrations, specialized entities, territorial collectivities and operators 2. Optimization of the use of units and resources
Prevention	3. Dissuade or prevent the occurrence of a CBRNE attack
Response (1)–Detection	4. Threat detection or detection of a CBRNE terrorist action
Response (2)–Protection of the population and potential targets	5. Protection of the population, sites and critical infrastructures
Response (3)–Intervention	6. Confronting a terrorist action, preventing the sequence of events 7. Responding to a real terrorist attack and conducting efficient and secure response actions 8. Assessment of the situation and mitigation of consequences 9. Caring for (potential) victims
Rehabilitation	10. Management of consequences to return back to normal as soon as possible

Fig. 9.1 Objectives of the state doctrine for the prevention and response to CBRNE terrorism

In case of a serious crisis such as a pandemic or bioterrorist event, while the President of the Republic and the Prime Minister are responsible for political and strategic actions, the Ministry of Interior takes charge of operational conduct of the response, the Ministry of Health remaining responsible for health issues. The Ministry of Interior can activate a decision-making interministerial crisis committee (CIC), involving representatives of cabinets or directorate of a number of ministries, including the Ministry of Health, as well as representatives of the National Defence General Secretariat and the Government Information Service. The Ministry of Health also activates the public health crisis centre. In addition, the Ministry of Foreign and European Affairs relies on a crisis centre permanently activated, which intervenes when a crisis threatens the security of nationals abroad or involves a humanitarian situation.

9.3.2 *Defence and Security Areas, a Key Level*

Governmental plans are adapted at the level of ministries, defence and security areas, and departments (one of the main administrative divisions in France). Defence and security areas, seven for metropolitan France and five overseas, constitute a key territorial division in terms of crisis management. The prefects for the defence and security areas (PZDS), coming under the authority of the Prime Minister and of each of the ministries, are responsible for the preparation and implementation of national security measures, notably those regarding civil security and crisis management, and supervising actions from regional and departmental prefects.

They have been granted broader competencies in 2010 to improve planning and crisis management capacities ("Décret n°2010-224, 4 March 2010"). Among other missions, they set direction and priorities, relying on an assessment of risks and potential effects of threats, and are tasked with the translation of governmental planning at the level of the area, ensuring the implementation at the departmental level is effective. They organize operational surveillance, are responsible for the coordination with military authorities regarding national and defence security measures, and coordinate civil security means and actions. Regarding this last mission, according to Article R.1311-3 of the Defence Code, they can involve public and private means, requisitioning them if necessary. Reference health institutions are designated in each defence and security area ("Décret n°2005-1764 du 30 décembre 2005 relatif à l'organisation du système de santé en cas de menace sanitaire grave et modifiant le Code de la santé publique").

The prefect for the defence and security area relies on an interministerial general staff (EMIZDS) and, in case of a crisis, can activate an operational centre at the level of the defence and security area (COZ), which ensures coordination of aid and rescue operations. A representative of the armed forces takes part in the EMIZDS. He relies on an inter-armed forces general staff for the defence area (EMIAZD), with close links with the EMIZDS, and organizes involvement of armed forces in civil defence missions.

9.3.3 Civil Security and the Involvement of the Armed Forces in the National Territory

Protection of the population and of the national territory is a priority. The French White Paper on defence and national security identifies a strategy involving both civil and military means. Armed forces must be able to contribute to the response, should a non-military crisis situation arise, whatever its nature. Law enforcement and civil security forces are first-responders, but armed forces can provide support, especially if public means are limited, inadequate, unavailable, or non-existent. Furthermore, the Ministry of Defence contributes directly to civil security and assistance, including in the context of public health threats, through civil security military units placed at the Ministry of Interior's disposal, as well as with the Paris Fire Brigade and Marseille Marine Fire Battalion, or the Army Health Service and its hospitals.

Armed forces can intervene within the national territory in several contexts:

- National security, including maintenance of law and order, armed forces participating in addition to law enforcement forces (police and gendarmerie);
- Civil security, which addresses "risk prevention whatever their nature, information, warning of populations, as well as protection of persons, possessions and environment against accidents, disasters and catastrophes by implementing

relevant measures and means under the responsibility of the State, "territorial collectivities" and other public or private persons" ("Loi n°2004-811 du 13 août 2004 de modernisation de la sécurité civile");
- Non-specific mission, such as making equipment available, with or without staff on secondment.

As explained in joint service concept CIA-0.7 n°163/DEF/CICDE/NP of 11 May 2007, on the national territory, among other missions, armed forces can contribute to the fight against terrorism, in particular international terrorism, the fight against arms trafficking, arms components and proliferation, the protection of sectors of vital importance, the protection of major events on the national territory, and aid and emergency relief for populations in a crisis situation.

Armed forces can assist following the appropriate administrative or legal requisition and, in specific cases, if there is otherwise a request for support. Administrative requisitions can occur in the context of maintenance of law and order, violation of public security in emergency cases, and intervening against terrorism or in the case of a major crisis on the national territory. Actions are then carried out under the responsibility of civil authority and under military command, in coordination with law enforcement authorities.

9.4 Legal Framework, Plans and Guidelines

9.4.1 Exceptional Situations and Serious Health Threats

Several dispositions govern exceptional situations which can call for the extension of powers granted to authorities and restrictions on fundamental liberties.

A decree by the Council of Ministries may proclaim a state of emergency under the Act n°55-385 of 3 April 1955, in the event of imminent danger arising from serious disturbances of public order or from events which by virtue of their nature and severity are deemed to be public disasters. Prorogation beyond 12 days may be authorized only by law. Comparing with the state of siege, civil authorities and not military ones are granted extended powers.

Article 36 of the 1958 French Constitution governs the state of siege, codified in Articles L.2121-1 to L.2121-8 of the Defence Code. Enacted by the Council of Ministers, it can be proclaimed only in case of imminent peril resulting either from a foreign war or an armed insurrection. Prorogation beyond 12 days may also be authorized only by law.

Besides, Article 16 of the Constitution extends the powers of the President of the Republic. It authorizes him to take measures required by the circumstances, "[w]hen the institutions of the Republic, the independence of the Nation, the integrity of its territory or the fulfillment of its international commitments are under serious and immediate threat, and when the proper functioning of the constitutional public powers is interrupted". The Constitution requires the President to consult the Prime Minister, Presidents of the Assemblies, and Constitutional Council (*Conseil constitutionnel*).

The latter then issues an advisory opinion that the President can disregard but which is made public. Constitution Act n°2008-724 of 23 July 2008 introduced democratic control on duration. After 30 days of exercising such powers, the president of one of the two assemblies, 60 Senators or 60 Members of the National Assembly can appeal to the Constitutional Council for it to consider whether the conditions laid in the first paragraph still apply. Its decision is publicly announced. After 60 days and at any moment thereafter, the Council carries out such an examination as matter of standard procedure.

Legislators went further regarding the specific issue of preparing the public health system for major health hazards. Law n°2004-806 of 9 August 2004 on public health policy created a new preliminary chapter regarding serious health threats in the Public Health Code. Law n°2007-294 of 5 March 2007 on the preparation of the health system to deal with large-scale health threats added other articles; this chapter became Chapter I of the new title dedicated to serious health threats.

Article L.3131-1 of this chapter states that "in the event of a major health hazard requiring emergency action, in particular a possible epidemic, the Minister for Health may, by order with justification and in the interests of public health, prescribe measures proportionate to the risk incurred and appropriate to circumstances of time and venue, in order to prevent and limit the consequences of the possible threats on the health of the population", and "[t]he Minister may empower the territorially competent representative of the State to take all the measures required for the implementation of these provisions", which implies the necessity to have an adequate articulation between the Ministry of Health and the Ministry of Interior. Article L.3110-2 rules that justifications of measures taken in implementation of the previous article must be periodically reviewed.

Considering these two articles, in a published opinion about ethical issues raised by a possible influenza pandemic, the National Consultative Ethics Committee for Health and Life Sciences (CCNE) draws attention to the risk of extending restrictions on fundamental liberties "beyond what is strictly required to contain the influenza pandemic, either because of a maximalist (and therefore inappropriate) conception of the precautionary principle or as a demagogic concession" [2].

The title about serious health threats also includes dispositions to protect health professionals from potential civil liability in carrying out their duties following decisions from the Ministry of Health accordingly, on the one hand, and makes provisions for compensation of potential victims, on the other hand. Some dispositions also relate to the constitution and organization of a health reserve corps.

9.4.2 Preparation and Response Plans

9.4.2.1 ORSEC Civil Emergency Plan

In France, the pre-hospital strategy in case of mass casualties relies on regulation and advanced medical posts, with a controlled evacuation in order to protect hospitals from massive influx. It thus differs from the "scoop and run" strategy where the patient is immediately taken to hospital.

Revised by law n°2004-811 of 13 August 2004, the ORSEC plan, adapted in each department and defence and security area, specifies the global organization of civil security response in the case of mass casualties and inventorying public and private resources which could be used. Some measures are generic, while others address specific risks and threats (e.g. white plans).

9.4.2.2 White Plans

Complementary with the previous plan, each public or private health institution has to develop a White Plan ("Circulaire n°DHOS/CGR/2006/401, 14 September 2006"), a crisis response plan in the case of a mass influx of patients or victims or in the case of an exceptional health crisis situation. They are also obliged to have an operational crisis cell responsible for alert and crisis management (Articles L.3110-7 to L.3110-10 of the Public Health Code). White Plans include a CBRN component. CBRN risk management takes into account the geographical location of health institutions as well as emerging risks.

White Plans are integrated in a "widened" White Plan, coordinating the public health system at the department level. It defines the role of health actors according to three types of scenarios: mass influx of victims with no risk of contamination, contaminated and contaminating victims, and evacuation of health medical institutions.

9.4.2.3 CBRN Threats and "Pirate" Plans

Vigipirate, a governmental plan of vigilance, prevention and protection, addresses terrorism and aims at protecting populations, institutions and infrastructures, as well as at preparing for response. It relies on a principle of shared responsibility and a permanent security posture, with the addition of graduated and flexible measures according to the national and international threat assessment. There are four colour-coded alert levels.

No indication of threat
Vague threat
Plausible threat
Highly plausible threat
Immediate threat of major attacks

This plan can be complemented by "Pirate" plans, focusing on specific threats. All these plans, elaborated under the responsibility of the SGDN (now SGDSN), result from an interministerial process.

The CBRN plan, which is classified, results from the merging of the Piratome (NR), Biotox (B) and Piratox (C) plans. The implementation of the whole plan or of part of it is not dependent on the Vigipirate alert level, but an alert level can involve the implementation of specific measures. The CBRN plan is regularly tested through exercises.

The plan specifies how to initiate the implementation of the plan, when necessary, and describes alert chains and responsibilities. Various situations are taken into account. It addresses for example issues such as contamination of the food chain, of a pharmaceutical chain or of the water network, as well as the receipt of a suspicious letter or parcel. It also considers events which could occur abroad, in order to be able to protect the national territory as well as to help French citizens which could be affected.

The CBRN plan is also complemented by other guidelines and plans such as:

- A document that details what procedure should be implemented in case of a suspicious letter, parcel, package or substances ("Circulaire n° 750/SGDSN/PSE/PPS, 18 February 2011"). To help avoid exceeding the analysis capacities, a specific cell (*Cellule nationale de Conseil* – CNC) has been created in the aftermath of the events in the United States in 2001. Its role is to contribute to a triage strategy and to help and counsel the department prefect.
- Specific guidelines regarding plague, anthrax and tularemia have been annexed. It deals in particular with: (1) Strategies of response, within three potential scenarios; (2) How to take charge of exposed individuals (on site, at home, at hospital), including evacuation and decontamination, as well as potential isolation; (3) How to transport specimens for the biological analysis, from the site of the bioterrorist attack to the laboratory; (4) How to plan for mass prophylaxis with antibiotics; (5) Environmental detection and decontamination; (6) How to take care of the deceased; and (7) Details and addresses for the Biotox-Piratox laboratories network. There is also a guide for toxins.
- A document addressing the consequences of a smallpox threat, specifying the strategy of response, including vaccination according to the number of exposed and geographic distribution, and the response organization. Mandatory vaccination was abrogated in 1984. However, Article L.3111-8 of the Public Health Code states that "in case of war, public disaster, epidemics or epidemic threat, anti-smallpox vaccination or re-vaccination can be made mandatory [...] for each person, whatever the age". Articles D.3111-19 to D.3111-21 give the specific details.
- A plan dedicated to the distribution of medicines which would be transported from national sites of stockpiling and would be distributed under the responsibility of a pharmacist, with the Minister of Health in charge of the coordination ("Circulaire du 20 mars 2003 relative à l'organisation de la distribution de médicaments dans le cadre d'une agression bio terroriste de grande ampleur").

Plans are periodically amended to take into account lessons learned from past crises and they are regularly tested through exercises at various levels.

9.4.2.4 Threat of Infectious Diseases and Specific Health Plans

Besides the smallpox governmental plan mentioned above, a number of other specific health plans address infectious diseases issues. They include the SARS and pandemic influenza national plans, as well as some plans, the implementation of which is required from prefects at the departmental level. They deal with the distribution of antibiotics (*Plan Fluoroquinolones*), drinking water, and air monitoring (*Plan Eau potable* and *Plan Air*).

9.5 Focus on Public Health Services

Public health services are key components, deeply involved at each stage, from preparation and prevention to early warning and crisis management. The cabinet of the Ministry of Health assesses propositions from public health agencies and issues decisions. The Senior Defence and Security Officer (HFDS) coordinates actions related to CBRN. In the case of a crisis, the Ministry can activate the public health crisis centre, which is in liaison with the Ministry of Interior's CIC and with health structures at territorial, national, European and international level.

The Ministry of Health includes a service dedicated to crisis situations, the Department of Public Health Emergencies (DUS). It relies on a number of public health agencies and on a laboratory network. The most relevant agencies in the context of an infectious disease crisis are the French National Institute for Public Health Surveillance (InVS), the French Health Products Safety Agency (AFSSAPS), and the Health Emergency Preparedness and Response Agency (EPRUS). Food safety and environmental issues are addressed by the French Agency for Food, Environmental and Occupational Health and Safety (ANSES).

9.5.1 Department of Public Health Emergencies (Département des Urgences Sanitaires – DUS)

This structure within the General Health Directorate, Ministry of Health, takes part in the preparation of the response to health risks and threats linked to natural events, outbreaks, technological accidents or terrorism acts, including bioterrorist events. It relies on a global integrated approach.

A key component, the DUS, develops policy and doctrine for the health reserve corps and prepares the response to serious health threats, including terrorist actions. It is responsible for the operational coordination of the response, including the operational management of emergency or health crisis situations. A unique point of entry for information relative to alerts, it gathers, analyses and registers information when national or international events occur. There is an operational centre for the reception and regulation of health and social emergencies (CORRUSS).

The DUS receives information from departmental and interregional institutions and from InVS. The DUS is also linked with other services dealing with crises, for example the Interdepartmental Operations Centre for Crisis Management (COGIC) of the Ministry of Interior or the French Joint Operations Planning and Command and Control Centre (CPCO) of the Ministry of Defence.

9.5.2 *French National Institute for Public Health Surveillance (Institut de Veille Sanitaire – INVS)*

InVS, the motto of which is "watch, monitor, alert", is responsible for continuous monitoring of the population's health status, health surveillance, health alerts, and assistance in health crisis management.

Surveillance of infectious diseases is one of the missions given to the Institute, tasked with identifying public health threats at an early stage, giving early warning, and providing information to decision-makers. It also monitors on-going events and does post-crisis evaluation in order to integrate lessons learned. In fiscal year 2010, the budget for the infectious disease surveillance programme amounted to EUR 21.2 million, representing 33% of the overall operating budget. The A(H1N1) influenza programme received an additional 2% [4].

The Institute uses specific as well as non-specific (syndromic) surveillance systems. Syndromic surveillance can be defined as the collection of non-statistical data on health trends, followed by their analysis and interpretation. Its objective is the early detection of health threats and real-time (or near real-time) health impact assessment of events. It has for example proven effective in the monitoring of infectious disease outbreaks such as gastrointestinal diseases, influenza, and viral meningitides, as well as cold spells or heat waves. This tool must be effectively integrated into the public health system [7]. It is intended to enhance and not replace other traditional approaches for epidemic detection.

Adapted to take into account bioterrorism (or even chemical or radiological terrorism), it could contribute to the early detection of a bioterrorist event, focusing on symptoms instead of confirmed diagnoses (detection through syndromic surveillance instead of through clinician reporting), thus reducing the delay between exposure and administration of a prophylactic or curative treatment (when available). It could also give information about the size, spread, and other characteristics of an outbreak after detection.

In France, the Syndromic Surveillance Programme was launched in 2004 by the InVS, following the consequences of the 2003 heat waves. Prior to that, the health surveillance and early warning systems were nearly entirely based on sentinel networks and mandatory declarations for a list of diseases. The methodology is based on use of retrospective and prospective studies. It implies defining specific criteria, like alert indicators and thresholds. Bioterrorism is one of the potential situations taken into account.

The French syndromic surveillance system, SurSaUD®, relies on three kinds of sources to collect data: emergency departments (OSCOUR® network), emergency general practitioners service (*SOS Médecins*) and, for mortality data, city registry offices. These three systems are entirely computerized and automated. The data are automatically collected daily, and then transmitted after encryption. This transfer respects the national patient confidentiality rules. For the sake of analysis, the following data are collected from the emergency departments: age, gender, zip-code, reason for emergency admission, and main medical diagnosis (based on the CIM10). The collected data must then be analyzed which relies on algorithms.

Evaluations are crucial to be able to demonstrate the utility of syndromic surveillance. However, they are difficult to carry out and specific criteria of evaluation must be defined [1]. The French system has, for example, been assessed in the context of the 2006 heat wave [3]. Almost all the data required for daily analysis were acquired. But one important observation was that it was not possible to use other data transmission methods other than internet, highlighting the necessity to develop solutions to be able to proceed even in case of a network failure. The authors also noted the study presented some limitations, as several parameters were not taken into account and the time period was limited as was the representativeness (with less than 40% of all emergency departments regional activity analyzed). They underlined the need to research and determine criteria which should be evaluated in other situations, as well as the possible necessity to confirm the results through other studies under the same weather conditions.

At the European level, the InVS coordinates Triple S – Syndromic Surveillance Survey and assessment towards guidelines for Europe – a 3-year project launched in 2010. Co-financed by the European Commission, it involves 24 organizations from 14 countries. Its objective is to assess existing European syndromic surveillance systems and will provide scientific and technical guidelines for the development of such systems. It aims at enhancing European capabilities regarding (near) real-time surveillance and monitoring in the context of expected or unexpected health-related events.

9.5.3 French Health Products Safety Agency (Agence Française de Sécurité Sanitaire des Produits de Santé – AFSSAPS)

Created in 1998, AFSSAPS's missions encompass scientific and medico-economic evaluation, laboratory control and advertising control, as well as inspections of industrial sites. It takes safety decisions concerning health products, from manufacturing to marketing, and coordinates monitoring activities once they are authorized. This includes the management and evaluation of biomedical research, to ensure protection for the people involved by assessing the safety and quality of products.

AFSSAPS contributes to preparedness and response against bioterrorism and emerging health threats by assessing therapies and publishing therapeutic guidelines. Factsheets for drug treatment protocols address anthrax, plague, tularaemia, brucellosis, viral hemorrhagic fevers, smallpox, botulinum toxin, Q fever, other bacterial infections, biological agents for which no specific or prophylactic treatment can be recommended, as well as the course of action in an emergency situation when the agent is not yet identified (available on the AFSSAPS website). It would be involved in crisis management regarding issues pertaining to medical countermeasures. It could for example need to issue temporary authorizations for use (ATU), which are exceptional procedures enabling the use of pharmaceutical products without a marketing authorization in France, outside the usual framework of a clinical trial (e.g. for smallpox vaccination). ATU can be granted for health products meant to treat, prevent, or diagnose serious or rare diseases, when no appropriate approved therapeutic alternative exists and when the efficiency and safety are presumed given current scientific knowledge of the product. Moreover, in this context, maintaining stockpiles means performing regular quality controls and has thus generated specific requirements in terms of laboratory activities.

At last, AFSSAPS contributes directly to biological safety and security. According to Article R.5139-1 of the Public Health Code, created by Decree n°2010-736 of 30 June 2010, it issues and manages authorizations regarding production, transport, importation, exportation, possession, supply, transfer, acquisition, and use of microorganisms and toxins. Article L.5139-1, modified by Ordinance n°2010-18 of 7 January 2010, specifies that these measures apply to microorganisms and toxins when their use could pose a risk for public health, as well as to products containing these agents.

9.5.4 Health Emergency Preparedness and Response Agency (Etablissement de Préparation et de Réponse Aux Urgences Sanitaires – EPRUS)

This specific structure was created in 2007 to improve preparation and response to health crises and is dedicated to the management of acquisition, production, imports, stockpiling and distribution of pharmaceutical products: it manages the French national stockpile of medical countermeasures ("Loi n°2007-294 du 5 mars 2007 relative à la préparation du système de santé à des menaces sanitaires de grande ampleur", "Décret n°2007-1273, 27 August 2007"). Its mission is to implement the crisis management strategies drafted by the General Health Directorate.

It also has to organize the health reserve corps, recruiting on a voluntary basis. It can be called when facing a situation of exception exceeding the usual capacities, in order to strengthen medical and social care structures. Reservists can be mobilized through a joint decree from the Ministries of Health and Interior. This corps is divided in two, with health professionals liable to be called up very quickly for intervention on national territory or abroad, and a pool including retired health professionals and medical and paramedical students for reinforcement in case of a long term serious health threat.

9.5.5 Biotox-Piratox Laboratories' Network

In 2003, in the aftermath of the anthrax letters event and the following hoaxes, a three-level laboratories network was created in order to deal with the consequences of a biological attack. The network includes civilian private and public laboratories, as well as military laboratories. A scientific council consisting of civilian and military experts meets monthly.

The network provides capacities in terms of biological or chemical toxicological analysis of environmental, veterinary or human samples. Laboratories can be involved in evaluating suspicious envelopes, parcels or substances; foul play against animals, plants, and especially the food chain, the water network, and the transport of biological agents; and victims in case of biological or chemical attacks. Achieving a better coordination and standardization of laboratory procedures implies a process of accreditation. Beyond detection and identification for crisis management, the objective is also to take into account forensics requirements and guarantee traceability with a procedure acceptable from a legal point of view (the sample constitutes evidence).

The first level of this network gathers many laboratories which have a role for screening and alert. They can collect and send samples, and ultimately proceed to a first analysis. The second level, which has a key role in the global system, is composed of reference laboratories and associated laboratories, designated in each defense area, and which have the capacities to identify some or all agents linked to bioterrorism. The last level is constituted by national reference laboratories; the BSL-4 laboratory is integrated in this level, as well as military laboratories such as the Centre d'Études du Bouchet (CEB) or the Centre de Recherche du Service de Santé des Armées (CRSSA).

9.6 Conclusions

From prevention to recovery, actions and response of stakeholders have a direct impact on the development and management of the crisis and its consequences. Proceeding to post-crisis assessments and sharing experiences, in order to enhance existing plans and procedures, is a crucial aim. The French plan against bioterrorism pre-dated the 2001 anthrax attacks, but these events, followed by numerous hoaxes, contributed to raise awareness and prompted a reassessment of existing measures. SARS outbreaks and influenza pandemic threats have also led to improvements in terms of biopreparedness.

Regardless of the nature of the potential crisis involving an infectious disease (natural, accidental or intentional), effective planning, preparedness training and efficient crisis communication have a determining impact on individual and societal resilience. In this perspective, one objective of the strategy developed in the pandemic influenza plan is indeed to organize and ensure continuity of Government action as well as of social and economic life. It is of importance to continue to adopt and adapt efficient institutional and business continuity plans to be able to face a public health crisis, and though there is a focus on critical infrastructure operators, all enterprises are encouraged to do so. But the key challenge remains to raise and maintain awareness not only of first-responders and operators but also of French citizens, as they are also key players, the reactions of whom may have a direct impact on the development and management of a crisis and its consequences.

References

1. Buehler J, Hopkins R, Overhage J, Sosin D, Tong V (2004) Framework for evaluating public health surveillance systems for early detection of outbreaks. MMWR 50(13):1–35
2. French National Ethics Committee for Health and Life Science (2009), Opinion n°106: Ethical issues raised by a possible influenza pandemic
3. Josseran L, Fouillet A, Caillère N, Brun-Ney D, Ilef D, Brucker G, Mediros H, Astagneau P (2010) Assessment of a syndromic surveillance system based on morbidity data: results from the Oscour network during heat wave. PLoS One 5(8):e11984
4. Institut de Veille Sanitaire (2011), Rapport Annuel 2010. Institut de Veille Sanitaire, Saint-Maurice, p 7
5. Mailles A, Alauzet C, Mock M, Garin-Bastuji B, Veran Y (2010) Cas groupés de charbon cutané humain en Moselle – Décembre 2008. Institut de Veille Sanitaire, Saint-Maurice
6. Mazuet C, Bouvet P, King LA, Popoff M (2011) Le botulisme humain en France, 2007–2009. BEH 6:49–53
7. Stoto M, Schonlau M, Mariano L (2004) Syndromic surveillance: is it worth the effort? Chance 17(1):19–24
8. Taylor T (2006) Safeguarding advances in the life sciences: The International Council for the Life Sciences is committed to becoming the authoritative source for identifying and managing biological risks. EMBO Rep 7:S61–S64

Chapter 10
Case Study – Germany

Christine Uhlenhaut, Lars Schaade, and Ernst-Jürgen Finke

Abstract Public health structures in Germany reflect the federal system: health care in general lies within the responsibility of the 16 constituent states and the federal government only acts if a state asks for assistance. There were no bioterror-related intentional releases of biological agents in Germany in recent years. The potentially devastating effects of such an incident require sound public health preparedness planning. The Basic Constitutional Law (*Grundgesetz*) does not allow the deployment of armed forces within Germany with some rare exceptions. However, there is a well-established civil-military cooperation. The Federal Armed Forces (*Bundeswehr*) are deployed in humanitarian and multinational UN or NATO crisis containment missions abroad, requiring adequate protection from pathogens and diseases endemic or enzootic to those regions. Both, the military and the civil public health system are complex structures that contain administrative, care giving, medical investigation, and research capabilities in order to cope with natural, accidental or intentional biological incidents.

10.1 Current Public Health Situation

Today, pathogens with significant public health impact in Germany are mostly bacteria and viruses. Compared to other geographic regions (with different climates and environmental conditions), parasites and fungi are only of minor importance.

The views expressed in this chapter reflect the views of E-J Finke and do not represent the official opinion of the Federal Ministry of Defence.

C. Uhlenhaut (✉) • L. Schaade
Centre for Biological Security, Robert Koch Institute, Berlin, Germany
e-mail: uhlenhautc@rki.de; schaadel@rki.de

E.-J. Finke
Scientific consultant in medical biological defence, Munich, Germany
e-mail: ernst.juergen.finke@online.de

I. Hunger et al. (eds.), *Biopreparedness and Public Health: Exploring Synergies*,
NATO Science for Peace and Security Series A: Chemistry and Biology,
DOI 10.1007/978-94-007-5273-3_10, © Springer Science+Business Media Dordrecht 2013

Biological agents such as prions and toxins are uncommon. Some of the most frequent infectious diseases are:

- Hepatitis B (former or current infection): about 7% of the general population [21].
- Hepatitis C: about 0.4% of the general population is seropositive [21].
- Influenza: on average, between 7,000 and 13,000 deaths per year due to seasonal influenza [30].
- HIV/AIDS: an estimated 73,000 persons currently infected, about 2,800 new infections per year [35].
- Tuberculosis: more than 7,000 cases per year [29].
- Food poisoning: about 200,000 cases are reported annually [29].
- Nosocomial infections: 400,000–600,000 cases annually, about 58,000 of whom require intensive care, resulting in an estimated 10,000–15,000 deaths [15, 16].

Although these and other infectious diseases are burdening the health care system significantly, the main causes of morbidity and mortality in Germany are consequences of chronic diseases. Amongst the ten most common causes of death, only pneumonia is directly linked to infection [45].

The relevant infectious diseases prevalent in Germany differ widely from agents that are perceived to be bioterrorism-relevant. A German assessment of biological agents that are considered to be of potential interest to bioterrorists mostly conforms to current international assessments, e.g. the CDC list [10], although there is no official German list of threat agents.[1] A comparison of the CDC list and the current German assessment shows some variations. Alphaviruses mentioned on the CDC list (such as eastern equine encephalitis virus and western equine encephalitis virus) are currently not considered to be agents of major concern in Germany. Another difference is the listing of food and water safety threats on the CDC list, such as *Salmonella*, *E. coli* and *Shigella* species. Furthermore, the CDC list includes emerging pathogens which are often omitted from bio-threat lists. In terms of public health response, those pathogens are covered by other mechanisms such as the International Health Regulations (IHR) and nationally by the German Protection against Infection Act (*Infektionsschutzgesetz*, IfSG).[2]

10.2 Risk Assessment for Potential Bioterrorism Agents

Compared to the impact of naturally occurring infectious diseases, currently most of the classical potential bioterrorism agents such as *B. anthracis*, botulinum neurotoxins, *Y. pestis*, Variola virus, *F. tularensis*, or viral hemorrhagic fever viruses are

[1] For selected highly pathogenic agents and toxins, the methods available in the Robert Koch-Institute for their detection, as well as the reference laboratories, see http://www.rki.de/DE/Content/Infekt/Biosicherheit/Diagnostik/Diagnostik-Detektion_node.html (accessed 21 May 2012).

[2] The law was adopted in 2000 and most recently updated on 28 July 2011; http://www.gesetze-im-internet.de/bundesrecht/ifsg/gesamt.pdf (accessed 29 August 2011).

not considered to pose an imminent risk in Germany. Rare cases of autochthonous as well as imported botulism and tularemia have been described [36]. In 2010, several cases of anthrax occurred among intravenous drug users [32–34]. Very few cases of viral hemorrhagic fevers – all of which had been imported – were treated in Germany [36]. No cases of plague were detected in recent years. Test systems are available for all currently relevant biological agents of either public health importance or those that are considered biothreat agents.

In principle, the same public health measures are required to control naturally occurring infectious diseases as well as diseases caused by the intentional release of pathogens or toxins (i.e. potential acts of bioterrorism or criminal acts). Consequently, most of the responding structures in Germany are identical. The legal basis for infection control in Germany is provided by the IfSG. It allows abrogating basic rights such as freedom of assembly or freedom of movement in order to control the spread of infections. This law also defines which diseases are notifiable (grouped into suspected cases, confirmed cases, and deaths) and sets the time frame for notification. There is a catch-all element implemented to also cover emerging pathogens or outbreaks of pathogens not explicitly mentioned in the law.

10.3 Public Health Structures and Regulations in the Civilian Sector

Germany is a federal state, and health care in general – including public health measures – is the responsibility of the 16 constituent states (*Bundesländer*). Each of these states has its own constitution and is largely autonomous. In case of notifiable diseases or pathogens, physicians on the local level initially notify the public health officer (*Amtsarzt*) and health agencies (*Gesundheitsämter*) of the municipality. However, the principle of subsidiarity applies and local authorities can ask for assistance. In case the local authorities are overwhelmed, they can request assistance from the county (*Landkreis*), the state, and the federal level. In cases or suspected cases of bioterrorism, the criminal investigations are performed by the Federal Criminal Police Office (*Bundeskriminalamt*, BKA).

On the federal level, the Federal Ministry of Health (*Bundesgesundheitsministerium*, BMG) is responsible for health policy, drafting bills, ordinances and administrative regulations. The BMG has five Higher Federal Authorities in its remit, the Robert Koch-Institute (RKI), the Paul-Ehrlich-Institute (PEI, Federal Institute for Vaccines and Biomedicines), the German Federal Institute of Medical Documentation and Information (DIMDI), the Federal Centre for Health Education (BZgA), and the Federal Institute for Drugs and Medical Devices (BfArM). Of these, the RKI is the central federal institution responsible for disease control and prevention. In a public health or bioterrorism emergency, the main responsibilities of the RKI are epidemiological and microbiological analysis as well as scientific support and counseling. An additional task is on-the-spot support on request of the federal state affected. The RKI is also the German authority providing information regarding the International Health Regulations (IHR) on infectious diseases via the German Joint

Information and Situation Centre (*Gemeinsames Melde- und Lagezentrum*, GMLZ) to the World Health Organization (WHO).

Within the RKI, the Centre for Biological Security (*Zentrum für Biologische Sicherheit*, ZBS) develops concepts for identifying bioterrorist attacks and diagnostic tools and capabilities for relevant pathogens. The centre is divided into the Federal Information Centre for Biological Security (*Informationsstelle des Bundes für Biologische Sicherheit*, IBBS) and six departments (ZBS1 to 6). ZBS1 works on highly pathogenic viruses, including developing diagnostic methods and strategies on how to combat and prevent infections with highly pathogenic viruses. Also affiliated to ZBS1 are two consultant laboratories: for tick-borne encephalitis and for orthopoxviruses. ZBS2 works on highly pathogenic bacteria, develops diagnostics for bacterial pathogens of high-risk groups, and also focuses on assuring the quality of diagnostics, e.g. through interlaboratory experiments (EQADeBa[3]). ZBS3 works on microbial toxins, including research on their pathogenesis. ZBS4 provides rapid diagnostics of relevant pathogens; mainly, this department focuses on different forms of electron microscopy. ZBS5 plans the building and setting up of a BSL-4 facility that is currently under construction. The newest addition, ZBS6, works on proteomics and spectroscopy of highly pathogenic organisms.

Other structures on the federal level are in the remit of the Federal Ministry of Food, Agriculture and Consumer Protection (BMELV). Here the Federal Institute for Risk Assessment (BfR) and the Federal Office of Consumer Protection and Food Safety (BVL) are responsible for a wide array of issues relating to food safety.

Several additional structures have been implemented as public health tools in a broader sense. Germany has 18 national reference centres that monitor important infectious diseases. In addition, there are currently 49 consultant laboratories to comprehensively cover a broad spectrum of pathogens. All of these centers and laboratories perform research but they also – to different degrees – develop detection assays, reference materials and guidelines for prevention, therapy and diagnostics [23]. In 2003, the German Working Group for the Management of Highly Contagious Diseases (*Ständige Arbeitsgemeinschaft der Kompetenz- und Behandlungszentren*, StAKoB) was founded. This unique network combines BLS-4 laboratory, clinical, and public health expertise. Its mission comprises the development of guidelines for treatment of highly contagious and life-threatening infections, development of training and education concepts, and definition of quality standards. Furthermore, StAKoB organizes personnel and material support as well as common exercises [17]. The current members of the StAKoB are:

- Berlin (center of competence and clinical treatment center).
- Frankfurt/Main (center of competence and clinical treatment center).
- Hamburg (center of competence and clinical treatment center).
- Leipzig (center of competence and clinical treatment center).

[3] Establishment of quality assurances for detection of highly pathogenic bacteria of potential bioterrorism risk, http://www.rki.de/EN/Content/Prevention/EQADeBa/EQADeBa_node.html (accessed 21 May 2012).

- Munich (center of competence and clinical treatment center).
- Saarbrücken (clinical treatment center).
- Stuttgart (center of competence and clinical treatment center).
- Würzburg (clinical treatment center).

In addition to legal structures such as the IfSG as well as administrative and research resources, Germany (federal and state level) has developed and agreed on two comprehensive strategic concepts that facilitate collaboration on the different federal levels in case of a large-scale biological emergency. One of these concepts details the necessary steps in response to a smallpox outbreak (*Bund-Länder-Rahmenkonzept zur Vorbereitung auf biologische Gefahrenlagen*) [37]. The second concept is the national influenza preparedness plan [31] which consists of three parts:

- Measures.
- Phase-oriented tasks and recommendations.
- Scientific context.

These two concepts are being permanently updated. Although they have been developed for specific pathogens, they can be considered excellent bases for controlling other public health emergencies.

In order to allocate the limited funding and research resources appropriately, prioritization tools are being developed for naturally occurring pathogens as well as for potential biothreat agents. In both cases prioritization has to be done comparatively and reproducibly although different factors need to be taken into account beyond the question of whether an outbreak is possibly related to an intentional release. For instance, socio-economic, political or cultural factors could play a very important role as to how an epidemic spreads or what the potential impact could be – these considerations can become very complex, especially in case of incidents with multinational or global dimensions. All of the ranking and prioritizing efforts have to be dynamic processes as the variables are constantly changing.

Two departments of the RKI develop tools for the assessment of human-pathogenic agents. IBBS is currently developing a matrix that combines scientific data, e.g. regarding pathogenicity or routes of transmission, with information obtained from alternative sources (e.g. intelligence services). The purpose of this matrix is to assess the threat potential of biological agents in respect to their malevolent use by terrorists or criminals. Ideally, this tool will enable an independent and reproducible threat and risk assessment for all biological agents for which relevant information is available.

The Department for Infectious Disease Epidemiology (*Abteilung für Infektionsepidemiologie*) developed a matrix for naturally occurring infectious diseases [3, 22]. The main purpose of this matrix is to identify pathogens with potentially severe public health consequences. Currently, 127 biological agents are scored and divided into four priority groups. The list contains not only bacteria and viruses but also prions, fungi, parasites and even an unidentified agent (unidentified agent causing Kawasaki syndrome). Only one of the "classical" biothreat agents scores in the highest priority group of this list pertaining to naturally occurring diseases (*Staphylococcus aureus* toxins). Several others are grouped in the second (e.g. *Brucella* spp., several hemorrhagic fever viruses, SARS corona virus and Variola virus) or the third priority group (e.g. *Bacillus anthracis*, different *Burkholderia* species, *Francisella tularensis*, *Vibrio cholerae* or *Yersinia pestis*), while several others are not listed at all (e.g. equine encephalitis viruses, Nipah virus, Japanese encephalitis virus). The fact that toxins such as abrin, ricin or saxitoxin are not mentioned reflects the fact that these are not transmissible pathogens.

Germany focuses not only on national preparedness but is greatly interested in maintaining and strengthening international plans and structures such as those provided by the European Centre for Disease Prevention and Control (ECDC), the WHO and other collaborative efforts such as the Global Health Security Initiative (GHSI). An important issue for controlling multinational disease outbreaks is the establishment of structures and tools for communication. In order to ensure ease of communication during a crisis, Germany conducts regional as well as national exercises and also participates in international exercises.

10.4 Health Care in the Armed Forces

The Basic Constitutional Law (*Grundgesetz*) prohibits deployment of armed forces within Germany, with some rare exceptions such as emergency relief in the case of a natural disaster. The civil-military cooperation (CIMIC) within Germany is based on the Law on Civil Protection and Disaster Relief (*Gesetz über den Zivilschutz und die Katastrophenhilfe des Bundes*). In addition, the Federal Armed Forces (*Bundeswehr*) are deployed in humanitarian aid and multinational UN or NATO crisis containment missions abroad. Currently, about 7,700 military personnel are deployed on various missions such as ISAF or KFOR [7]. Some of these missions take place in tropical or subtropical areas and thus soldiers might contract not only diseases endemic in Germany but also pathogens and parasites endemic in these regions. Many of these pathogens are considered to be biological agents that may potentially be misused by terrorist or militant groups.

The health care for soldiers is the responsibility of the Chief of Staff of the Medical Service (*Inspekteur des Sanitätsdienstes der Bundeswehr*, InspSan) at the Federal Ministry of Defence (*Bundesministerium für Verteidigung*, BMVg). The implementation of public-legal tasks in the fields of hygiene and infection protection is the mission of the *Bundeswehr* Medical Office (*Sanitätsamt der Bundeswehr*, SanABw) and the medical commands (*Sanitätskommandos*, SanKdo). However, these structures are currently undergoing organizational changes due to the structural reform of the *Bundeswehr*.

Disease surveillance, prevention and control, and hygiene supervision are the responsibility of special departments of health and veterinary services at the SanABw and at the medical commands. Laboratory and investigational support is provided by the *Bundeswehr* Central Institutes of Medical Service (Zentrale Institute des Sanitätsdienstes der Bundeswehr, ZInstSanBw) in Coblenz, Kiel and Munich (comparable to the civilian country health investigation offices), the special branch of tropical medicine of the *Bundeswehr* at the Bernhard Nocht Institute in Hamburg, and the *Bundeswehr* Institute of Microbiology (*Institut für Mikrobiologie der Bundeswehr*, InstMikroBioBw), which was established in 2002 in Munich [8].

In case of outbreaks of communicable diseases in military communities, inspection, sampling, epidemiological and laboratory investigations, as well as anti-epidemic countermeasures will be performed by fact-finding or epidemiological investigation teams and specialists of the *Bundeswehr* health and veterinary services using medical intelligence. In parallel, military practitioners, clinicians and microbiological laboratories report diseases or notifiable pathogens:

- to the local public health officers and health agencies as required by the IfSG.
- to the senior hygienists of the departments of health service at regional medical commands, who notifies the SanABw according to the military chain of command [8].

The SanABw sends summary notifications to the staff department of the BMVg and to the RKI. Notifications from deployed *Bundeswehr* contingents are passed through a special military chain to the Operations Command (*Einsatzführungskommando*) in Germany, the responsible medical commands, and the SanABw for final epidemiological risk assessment.

Medical biological defence lies with the responsibility of the Bundeswehr Medical Service with the aim to protect, contain and restore the health of soldiers under threat or exposure with biological warfare or related agents, to control biological environments and to investigate and verify a deliberate use of biological agents in cooperation with the Bundeswehr NBC troops and the Military Research Institute for Protective Technologies and NBC Protection (*Wehrwissenschaftliches Institut für Schutztechnologien und ABC-Schutz*, WIS) in Munster.

Taking into account factors such as growing international terrorism and weaknesses of international disarmament control mechanisms in preventing the development and production of biological weapons, the NATO alliance leaders at their Summit in Prague 2002 under the Prague Capabilities Commitments agreed to develop and improve the capabilities to cope with biological threats [25]. These requirements have been implemented in May 2003 by the new Defence Policy Guidelines (*Verteidigungspolitische Richtlinien*) widening the range of the *Bundeswehr* to multinational operations in order to cope with crises and conflicts, to support NATO partners also under CBRN conditions and to assist in disasters [9]. In order to improve the preparedness of allied armed forces against emergencies due to natural epidemics or acts of bioterrorism, the Committee of the Chiefs of Military Medical Services in NATO (COMEDS) decided in Vilnius 2008 to build a multinational Deployment Health Surveillance Capability (DHSC) which was established in January 2010 at the *Bundeswehr* Medical Office in Munich [1]. Its main task will be the near-real-time epidemiological monitoring and symptoms-based detection of outbreaks during missions. Currently, international terrorism and proliferation of dual-use know how and weapons of mass destruction are regarded as the most significant threats (White Book on security policy of Germany and future of *Bundeswehr*) [6].

To ensure the availability of adequate resources, the Department for Medical NBC Defence Task Force at the SanABw with Medical Biological Reconnaissance Teams (MBRT) of the affiliated *Bundeswehr* Institute of Microbiology were established in 2003. In 2004, the Action Plan "Civilian crisis prevention, conflict resolution and consolidation of peace" and a new "Conception of the *Bundeswehr*" [9] were enacted. In 2005, the special concept for Medical NBC Defence (*Fachkonzept Medizinischer ABC-Schutz*), first introduced in 1997, was adapted. The spectrum as well as the ranking of potential biothreat agents applied here is variable and results from a dynamic risk assessment process by different expert panels, e.g. the Australia group [2], CDC (category A, B and C agents) or the NATO Biomedical Advisory Committee (BioMedAC Expert Panel) of the COMEDS [25].

The *Bundeswehr* Institute of Microbiology is one of the scientific reach-back capabilities of the BMVg in the case of natural and intentional biological emergencies and takes scientific leadership for special diagnostics as well as for applied research and development [8]. It conducts integrated research in cooperation with military (NATO, Partnership for Peace) and civilian scientific and commercial partners in Germany and internationally, using different scientific networks and cooperative biological research programmes, e.g. of the European Defence Agency (EDA). In 2011, the *Bundeswehr* Institute of Microbiology became a partner of the Centre for Infection Medicine Munich (*Zentrum für Infektionsmedizin München*) of the German Centre for Infection Research (*Deutsches Zentrum für Infektionsforschung*) [5].

The *Bundeswehr* Institute of Microbiology provides special advice, concepts, guidelines, instructions, procedures, and measures to the Chief of Medical Service and other military or civilian stakeholders. The institute has a Central Diagnostic Laboratory (CDL) at its disposal, comprising four research departments with specialized laboratories (among them a BSL-3 laboratory and national Consultant Laboratories for tularemia and brucellosis), and the Department of Medical Biological Reconnaissance and Verification with MBRTs.

The CDL implements a broad array of cultural, molecular-biological and immunological diagnostics. It uses in-house assays developed, validated and certified by the research departments of the institute according to the requirements of the European Directive on in vitro diagnostic medical devices, permitting the identification, differentiation and typing of most of the bacterial and viral agents listed by the CDC. At present, an analysis list and request forms are offered to all medical facilities of the *Bundeswehr*, but can also be obtained on request by civilian customers. These diagnostic capabilities were developed by the *Bundeswehr* Institute of Microbiology within the framework of a long-term applied research programme of the BMVg on diagnosis, pathogenesis, immunology, epidemiology and microbial forensics of potential biothreat agents and related health disorders. The institute's laboratories take part in internal and external quality assurance processes at national and international level by participation in military and civilian inter-laboratory proficiency and round-robin tests, e.g. INSTAND, EQADeBa, QCMD, and contribute to the standardization of diagnostics [26, 39].

In case of unusual outbreaks of diseases or suspected acts of bioterrorism, in addition to notification as required by IfSG and IHR, the Medical CBRN Defence

Department of SanABw can deploy its Medical NBC Task Force with MBRTs and specialists of the *Bundeswehr* Institute of Microbiology communicating by telemedicine. The MBRTs offer rapidly deployable modular field laboratories with equipment for personal protection, decontamination, sample collection and secure transportation of specimens as well as rapid detection and identification techniques, validated SOPs for different deployment scenarios and trained multi-disciplinary staff [38]. This ensures the interoperability within NATO as required by NATO standardization agreements (NATO STANAG) for Rapidly Deployable Outbreak Investigation Teams (RDOIT), prompt investigation of suspicious outbreaks, as well as special medical advice and information for commanders and medical authorities [25, 46]. The teams assist in the prophylaxis and clinical management as well as in infection prevention and control, including force protection, safety of health care workers and waste disposal. In case of suspected acts of bioterrorism or violations of the BTWC, MBRTs also sample specimens for laboratory verification at the *Bundeswehr* Institute of Microbiology according NATO standards. Consequently, the teams have been evaluated by multinational field exercises [38].

Within this context, deployable medical reconnaissance and special diagnostic capabilities of the *Bundeswehr* Institute of Microbiology have been offered already within CIMIC to support other federal departments in security measures and medical care during public events in Germany. They have also assisted civilian institutions (e.g. health agencies) to investigate unusual outbreaks caused by *Francisella tularensis holarctica* near Göttingen in 2004 [44] and Darmstadt in 2006 [20], or by Puumala virus in Lower Bavaria in 2004 [24]. The support provided included monitoring natural foci in order to assess infection risks and to distinguish epidemic/epizootic "background signals" from zoonoses (tick borne encephalitis, tularemia, rickettsial and hanta virus diseases) in training and mission areas of the *Bundeswehr*.

Since the 1990s, specialists of the *Bundeswehr* Institute of Microbiology and its predecessor, the former Institute of Microbiology of the *Bundeswehr* Medical Academy (*Sanitätsakademie der Bundeswehr*) Munich, have been participating in different expert or working groups and scientific networks of NATO (e.g. Biological Medical Advisory Council), WHO (e.g. Smallpox Advisory Committee on Variola Virus Research), EU (European Networks of Imported Viral Diseases and BSL-4 Laboratories, European Defence Agency). The institute has assisted in outbreak investigations or risk assessment on request by:

- the WHO/GOARN in Kosovo in 2000 on tularemia, and in 2008 on Crimean Congo hemorrhagic fever [19, 47].
- the Pasteur Institute Madagascar since 1999 on plague [27].
- the Democratic Republic of Congo since 2001 on monkey pox, and in 2003 on Ebola hemorrhagic fever [18, 28].
- the United Arab Emirates since 2004 on glanders [41].
- and the Netherlands in 2010 on Q fever.

Already prior to the events of 9/11 and Amerithrax in the USA and especially thereafter, the BMVg has been supporting the civilian health service in order to improve the preparedness against natural or intentional biological threats. Between 2000 and 2006 the civilian-military specialist group "Epidemics Protection-CIMIC" and the interdisciplinary expert group "Biological Threats" at the RKI developed concepts for the management of life-threatening imported infectious diseases with a national network of competence and treatment centres (see section on StAKoB above), a draft concept for national influenza pandemic preparedness, and handbooks on the management of dangerous biological events as well as guidelines for disaster, emergency and public health services [4, 13, 14, 17, 30, 31, 35–37]. These concepts were adapted to the special requirements of the medical support of soldiers deployed in Germany or abroad, resulting e.g. in the influenza pandemic planning and *Bundeswehr* Hospital Alert and Emergency Plans.

The special advice of the *Bundeswehr* Institute of Microbiology on medical biological defence is available on demand via the BMVg also for other federal departments and authorities, public health agencies, civilian scientific institutions, and medical societies in the form of assessments, training courses, workshops, or conferences, e.g. at the *Bundeswehr* Medical Academy, or at the Academy of Crisis Management, Emergency Planning and Civil Protection (*Akademie für Krisenmanagement, Notfallplanung und Zivilschutz*). Relevant expertise on medical biological defence has been introduced in special publications, guidelines and handbooks covering e.g. aspects of disaster, emergency or infection medicine [12, 40, 42], and in NATO Advanced Research Workshops [11, 43].

Since 1994, on behalf of the BMVg, the *Bundeswehr* Institute of Microbiology holds the international Medical Biological Defence conferences at the *Bundeswehr* Medical Academy in Munich almost every year and since 2007 biannually. The conference has become a successful international event in this special field. It offers civilian and military researchers as well as medical and political stakeholders from all over the world a scientific forum to exchange actual assessments of biological risks and threats, perspectives and developments in diagnosis, prevention, treatment, and anti-epidemic management of diseases caused by pathogens of concern, and reconnaissance and verification of unusual events. Here, the results of the full range of applied research and development of the BMVg at the *Bundeswehr* Institute of Microbiology and the WIS are presented. This conference represents an example of an important confidence-building measure of Germany within the framework of the BTWC.

10.5 Conclusion

The current assessment of the potential public health impact of naturally occurring versus intentionally caused infectious diseases comes to the conclusion that intentional release is not likely at this time. However, due to the potential magnitude of either event it is crucial to keep up with scientific developments and findings of security agencies. It is equally important to strengthen public health structures, to implement communication structures and to identify vulnerabilities ahead of time.

References

1. Allert B (2011) NATO Disease Surveillance Seminar. Medical Corps International Forum (mcif) 3./4.-2011, 70–71. http://www.mci-forum.com/media/issue/38/mcif_3_2011.pdf. Accessed 21 Dec 2011
2. Australia Group (2011). http://australiagroup.net/en/index.html. Accessed 21 Dec 2011
3. Balabanova Y, Gilsdorf A, Buda S, Burger R et al (2011) Communicable diseases prioritized for surveillance and epidemiological research: results of a standardized prioritization procedure in Germany. PLoS One 6:e25691
4. BBK (2007) Handbuch für den Bevölkerungsschutz: Biologische Gefahrenlagen, and Biologische Gefahren II. Entscheidungshilfen zu medizinisch angemessenen Vorgehensweisen in einer B-Gefahrenlage, Bonn
5. BMBF (2011) http://www.bmbf.de/de/16544.php. Accessed 21 Dec 2011
6. Bundeswehr (2006) Weißbuch 2006. http://www.bmvg.de/resource/resource/MzEzNTM4MmUzMzMyMmUzMTM1MzMyZTM2MzEzMDMwMzAzMDMwMzAzMDY3NmE2ODY1NmQ2NzY4MzEyMDIwMjAyMDIw/WB_2006_dt_mB.pdf. Accessed 20 May 2012
7. Bundeswehr (2011a) Numbers of German personnel deployed on the various missions. http://www.bmvg.de/portal/a/bmvg/!ut/p/c4/NY1BC4JAFIT_0T6tCOpWhNClLlHZZVndpz7SXXn7VJB-fCvRDMzAfIeBF0Q7M1JthLwzLTwhL2lfTKroxloFKhvkBklC71sSei skF4zMuhqQ-tUWnKyaM_QMoM8aVdTE4i2HChuGxnFhUpXcoSwo6oZg1G_Gses_SLmRgjkSRhTxJT8ckTf5KP9vNPbutNuvd-ZJdoe-6wxeABEql/. Accessed 21 Dec 2011
8. Bundeswehr (2011b) http://www.sanitaetsdienst-bundeswehr.de/portal/a/sanitaetsdienst/. Accessed 21 Dec 2011)
9. Bundeswehr (2011c) http://www.bmvg.de/portal/a/bmvg/. Accessed 21 Dec 2011
10. CDC (2011) Bioterrorism agents/diseases. http://www.bt.cdc.gov/agent/agentlist.asp. Accessed 22 Oct 2011
11. Dando M, Pearson G, Kriz B (eds) (2001) Scientific and technical means of distinguishing between natural and other outbreaks of diseases. NATO science series. 1. Disarmament technologies, vol 35. Kluwer Academic Publishers, Dordrecht/Boston/London
12. Darai G, Handermann M, Sonntag HG, Zöller L (eds) (2011) Lexikon der Infektionskrankheiten des Menschen – Erreger, Symptome, Diagnose, Therapie und Prophylaxe. Springer, Berlin
13. Fock R, Koch U, Finke EJ, Niedrig M et al (2000) Schutz vor lebensbedrohenden importierten Infektionskrankheiten: Strukturelle Erfordernisse bei der Behandlung und anti-epidemische Maßnahmen. Bundesgesundheitsbl Gesundheitsforsch Gesundheitsschutz 42:891–899
14. Fock R, Bergmann H, Bussmann H et al (2002) Influenza pandemic: preparedness planning in Germany. Eurosurveillance 7(1):1–5
15. Gastmeier P, Geffers C (2008) Nosokomiale Infektionen in Deutschland: Wieviel gibt es wirklich? Eine Schätzung für das Jahr 2006. Dtsch Med Wochenschr 133:1111–1115
16. Geffers C, Gastmeier P (2011) Nosocomial infections and multidrug-resistant organisms in Germany: epidemiological data from KISS (The Hospital Infection Surveillance System). Dtsch Arztebl Int 108:87–93
17. Gottschalk R, Grunewald T, Biederbick W (2009) Aufgaben und Funktion der Ständigen Arbeitsgemeinschaft der Kompetenz- und Behandlungszentren für hochkontagiöse, lebensbedrohliche Erkrankungen. Bundesgesundheitsblatt Gesundheitsforschung Gesundheitsschutz 52:214–218
18. Grolla A, Lucht A, Dick D, Strong JE et al (2005) Laboratory diagnosis of Ebola and Marburg hemorrhagic fever. Bull Soc Pathol Exot 98:205–209
19. Grunow R, Finke EJ (2002) A procedure for differentiating between the intentional release of biological warfare agents and natural outbreaks of disease: its use in analyzing the tularemia outbreak in Kosovo in 1999 and 2000. Clin Microbiol Infect 8:510–521
20. Hauri AM, Hofstetter I, Seibold E, Kaysser P et al (2010) Investigating an airborne tularemia outbreak, Germany. Emerg Infect Dis 16:238–243
21. Hellenbrand W (2003) Neu und vermehrt auftretende Infektionskrankheiten. Gesundheitsberichterstattung des Bundes No. 18. Robert Koch Institute, Berlin

22. Krause G (2008) How can infectious diseases be prioritized in public health? A standardized prioritization scheme for discussion. EMBO Rep 9(Suppl 1):S22–S27
23. Laude G, Ammon A (2005) Die Nationalen Referenzzentren und Konsiliarlaboratorien. Bedeutung und Aufgaben. Bundesgesundheitsblatt Gesundheitsforschung Gesundheitsschutz 48:998–1004
24. Mertens M, Wölfel R, Ullrich K, Yoshimatsu K et al (2009) Seroepidemiological study in a Puumala virus outbreak area in South-East Germany. Med Microbiol Immunol 198:83–91
25. NATO (2011) http://www.nato.int/cps/en/natolive/topics_50087.htm. Accessed 21 Dec 2011
26. Podbielski A, Herrmann M, Kniehl E, Mauch H (eds) (2008) Qualitätsstandards in der mikrobiologisch-infektiologischen Diagnostik. MiQ 26. Hochpathogene Erreger, Biologische Kampfstoffe, Teil I-IV. Elsevier, Munich
27. Riem J, Scholz HC, Rahalison L, Pfeffer M et al (2010) Validation von Real-time-PCR-Verfahren zur Detektion/zum Nachweis von Yersina pestis in klinischen Untersuchungsmaterialien von Patienten mit Verdacht auf Beulenpest. Wehrmed Monatsschr 54(3):79–82
28. Rimoin AW, Kisalu N, Kebela-Ilunga B, Mukaba T et al (2007) Endemic human monkey pox, Democratic Republic of Congo, 2001–2004. Emerg Infect Dis 13:934–937
29. RKI (2006) Gesundheit in Deutschland. http://www.gbe-bund.de/gbe10/owards.prc_show_pdf?p_id=9965&p_sprache=D. Accessed 20 May 2012
30. RKI (2007a) Epidemiologisches Bulletin 35/2007. http://www.rki.de/DE/Content/Infekt/EpidBull/Archiv/2007/Ausgabenlinks/35_07.pdf?__blob=publicationFile. Accessed 20 May 2012
31. RKI (2007b) Nationaler Influenzapandemieplan. http://www.rki.de/DE/Content/InfAZ/I/Influenza/Influenzapandemieplan.html. Accessed 21 May 2012
32. RKI (2010a) Epidemiologisches Bulletin 2/2010. http://edoc.rki.de/documents/rki_fv/re8UuoNfJNfHM/PDF/28fNLdaeJg1u_02.pdf. Accessed 21 May 2012
33. RKI (2010b) Epidemiologisches Bulletin 14/2010. http://edoc.rki.de/documents/rki_fv/reEgI2XxiZUCY/PDF/28woZVMa8dwJWY.pdf. Accessed 21 May 2012
34. RKI (2010c) Epidemiologisches Bulletin 49/2010. http://edoc.rki.de/documents/rki_fv/reflqZx2NGF02/PDF/202B0afYnEUn2.pdf. Accessed 21 May 2012
35. RKI (2011a) Epidemiologisches Bulletin 46/2011. http://edoc.rki.de/documents/rki_fv/reHrW6KJGUCQ/PDF/271mGoLnaBmkQ.pdf. Accessed 21 May 2012
36. RKI (2011b) Infektionsepidemiologisches Jahrbuch meldepflichtiger Krankheiten für 2010. http://www.rki.de/DE/Content/Infekt/Jahrbuch/Jahrbuch_2010.pdf?__blob=publicationFile. Accessed 21 May 2012
37. RKI (2011c) Das Bund-Länder-Rahmenkonzept zu notwendigen fachlichen Vorbereitungen und Maßnahmen zur Seuchenbekämpfung nach bioterroristischen Anschlägen. Teil: Pocken. http://www.rki.de/DE/Content/Infekt/Biosicherheit/Schutzmassnahmen/Beispiel_Pocken/beispiel-pocken_node.html. Accessed 21 May 2011
38. Schmidt S, Wölfel R, Mossbrugger I, Zöller L (2011) State-of-the-art procedures for in-the-field and stationary laboratory diagnosis of biological agents. Suppl. to mcif 3./4-2011: CHALLENGE: International Forum for Medical Biological Defence. 1/2001 19–22
39. Schmoldt S, Thoma BR, Wölfel R, Georgi E, et al (2011) Coping with quality management requirements in the laboratory diagnosis of biothreat agents and agent-related health disorders. Medical Biological Defense Conference 2011, Munich, 25–28 October 2011, Abstract 0080, in: Medical Corps International Forum 4/4 (2011), Suppl. 30
40. Scholz GJ, Sefrin P, Böttiger BW, Dörges V, et al (eds) (2012) Notfallmedizin, in preparation
41. Scholz HC, Joseph M, Tomaso H, Dahouk A et al (2006) Detection of the reemerging of Burkholderia mallei in a recent outbreak of glanders in the United Arabic Emirates by a newly developed fliP-based polymerase chain reaction assay. Diagn Microbiol Infect Dis 54:241–247
42. Schutzkommission BMI (ed) (2010) Katastrophenmedizin Leitfaden für die ärztliche Versorgung im Katastrophenfall, München
43. Sohns T, Voicu VA (eds) (1999) NBC risks – current capabilities and future perspectives for protection. NATO science series. 1. Disarmament technologies Vol. 25. Kluwer Academic Publishers, Dordrecht/Boston/London

44. Splettstoesser WD, Matz-Rensing K, Seibold E, Tomaso H et al (2007) Re-emergence of Francisella tularensis in Germany: fatal tularaemia in a colony of semi-free-living marmosets (*Callithrix jacchus*). Epidemiol Infect 135:1256–1265
45. Statistisches Bundesamt (2010) Statistisches Jahrbuch 2010. https://www.destatis.de/DE/Publikationen/StatistischesJahrbuch/StatistischesJahrbuch2010.pdf?__blob=publicationFile. Accessed 11 May 2011
46. Thibault, FM (2011) RDOIT: the NATO toolbox for suspect outbreak investigation. Medical Biodefence Conference 2011, Munich, 25–28 October 2011, in: Medical Corps International Forum 4/4-2011/Supplement 15
47. Wölfel R, Paweska JT, Petersen N, Grobbelaar AA et al (2009) Low-density macroarray for rapid detection of and identification of Crimean-Congo hemorrhagic fever virus. J Clin Microbiol 47:1025–1030

Chapter 11
Case Study – Greece

Nikolaos V. Zaras

Abstract Biological terrorism and the need for biological defence is a relatively new concept for Greece. Although defence against weaponized pathogens was part of CBRN training in the military, it was the 9/11 massacre followed by the anthrax letters horror that triggered a more active involvement of the Greek public health sector. In that historical moment a third bullet was added to the already existing disease outbreak classification – naturally, accidental and now deliberate. These incidents and the subsequent 2004 Olympic Games in Athens drove the Greek government to focus on biodefence and revise existing civil emergency planning by inclusion of new emerging threats.

11.1 Introduction

Naturally occurring or accidental outbreaks of a disease usually take place in both urban and country environments. Big cities are usually the targets of bioterrorism due to the high density of population resulting in both physical and psychological casualties.

If the disease does not start from one's own country then early warning might be possible, leading to preventive measures all the way from the borders into the community. The H1N1 virus pandemic is an example of this globalization of medical information that is useful to both countries and citizens.

N.V. Zaras (✉)
Special Joint CBRN Company, Hellenic Army, Athens, Greece
e-mail: nikzaras@yahoo.gr

I. Hunger et al. (eds.), *Biopreparedness and Public Health: Exploring Synergies*, NATO Science for Peace and Security Series A: Chemistry and Biology,
DOI 10.1007/978-94-007-5273-3_11,

Table 11.1 Distribution of specific diseases in Greek citizens and immigrants (2010)

	Declared cases among			
Disease	Immigrants (number)	Immigrants (percentage)	Greeks (number)	Greeks (percentage)
Malaria	38	84.44	7	15.56
Tuberculosis	229	46.93	259	53.07
Shigellosis	1	3.03	32	96.97
Hepatitis A	5	8.47	54	91.53
Hepatitis B	12	35.29	22	64.71
Typhoid fever	6	60.0	4	40.00
Brucellosis	11	11.34	86	88.66

Source: Epidemiological Surveillance System, CDCP

11.2 Main Public Health Threats

One important parameter of the epidemiology of infectious diseases is the movement of the populace either for professional, recreational or immigration reasons. In the past, moving from one location to another, even within the same country borders, took considerable time. In modern times, usually less than 24 h is needed to cross the world. We witnessed the contribution of faster travel to the spread of disease recently during the 2010 flu pandemic. Apart from the legal movement of a population, mass illegal immigration also poses a significant problem in certain parts of the world – e.g. in Greece – in relation to the spread of a disease or re-emergence of old diseases like malaria or tuberculosis. The geographical location of Greece and its porous borders due to the significant coastline make it an attractive destination for those seeking a better living environment or as a way to enter other EU countries as a final destination.

Greece receives a considerable number of tourists annually that exceeds its own population. Greeks also travel globally for the reasons mentioned above. This constant movement of a populace makes epidemiologic surveillance and disease prevention extremely difficult.

The reality of disease transmission as a result of immigration and travel is reflected below in the results from the Hellenic Centre for Disease Control and Prevention (CDCP) [2] and various relevant NGOs addressing the health status of immigrants and transmission of old and new infectious diseases. The percentage of declared cases of specific diseases attributed to Greek citizens and immigrants is shown in Table 11.1.

11.3 Bioterrorism as a Potential Threat

Timely information is crucial when it comes to a natural or accidental outbreak of a disease. This information might be beneficial to laboratory or institution workers or the population that needs to be protected. Of course, in most cases, basic hygiene measures (personal or collective, at home or in a wider infrastructure such as schools) can prevent these diseases.

Defence against a deliberate outbreak of a disease requires intelligence. This type of medical intelligence is attributed to national intelligence service both civilian and military. Usually international collaboration is mandatory when weaponized pathogens are the problem.

Risk identification and assessment contribute to national defence as well. It is a continuous process dealing with both the deliberate and non-deliberate forms of disease outbreaks. Internal (sanitary institutions, police reports, etc.) and external (neighboring countries, World Health Organization, EU public health surveillance systems, etc.) hints can assist experts to perform a risk assessment leading to an alert of the public health system.

Current geopolitical instability and turmoil in our own region combined with the existing direct and indirect, overt and covert threats against Western societies make bioterrorism attacks a potential risk.

Production of biological weapons is both easy and cost effective. Of course we must discriminate between the production and weaponization of pathogens that is not as easy and needs specialized equipment. Pathogen production does not require large factories and existing facilities in commercial infrastructure (food industry, drug industry) can be used for this purpose. On a smaller scale, pathogens can be cultivated in small laboratories or mobile caravans similar to those used to produce illegal drugs. Identification of such illegal laboratories is very difficult. Viral pathogens are more difficult to produce as compared to bacteria and also need some extra precautions and equipment.

Large quantities of biological weapons can still be produced in a short period of time (days or weeks) in small laboratories. According to Kathleen C. Bailey, former Assistant Director, Office for Disarmament and Armaments Control, who visited many biotechnology and pharmacology companies, a complete biolab requires no more than a room of 4.5 m × 4.5 m and a budget of USD 15,000 for supplies [1]. In such a room, trillions of bacteria can be quickly produced with low risk and with minimum personal protection equipment such as a gas mask and a plastic suit over clothing.

Difficulties relevant to the production of biological weapons include:

- Difficulties in the protection of workers at all levels of production, transportation, and final dispersal of biological weapons;
- Low level of training and expertise can lead to accidents and exposure to pathogens;
- Vaccination of those involved is not always protective/effective;
- Controlling the quality and quantity of produced material is difficult;
- Dispersion is not without problems since dispersal device explosives, UV exposure, or weather conditions such as rain or drying may have negative effects on pathogens or spores;
- Storage of pathogens poses additional problems; specific conditions are required to maintain the efficacy, and it is difficult to maintain them in a form ready for dispersion over long periods of time.

11.4 Preparedness and Response to Health Emergencies in Greece

Key stakeholders in public health preparedness and response systems are:

- General Secretariat of Civil Protection (GSCP) [3] – Organization under the Ministry of Citizen Protection [5] having the overall responsibility for the protection of the population against all disasters [4], either natural (earthquakes, wildfires, floods, landslides, severe weather phenomena etc.), technological, or deliberate (large scale terrorist attacks – CBRN agents release included).
- Centre for Disease Control and Prevention (CDCP) – Organization aiming to protect and promote public health by employing a national strategy for the prevention of disease spread. CDCP is responsible for the surveillance of epidemics, running infectious disease cells at hospitals throughout the country, management of public health hazards, and provision of public guidelines in case a public hazard emerges. It is under the control and funding of the Ministry of Health and Social Solidarity [6] operating on a 24/7 basis.
- First Aid National Centre (EKAB) – Organization supporting medical transportation of casualties to state medical facilities.
- Hellenic Police, Hellenic Fire Service, and National Defence General Staff – Entities supporting GSCP's general emergency plan under the name "Xenocrates".

11.4.1 Epidemiologic Monitoring in Greece

Epidemiologic monitoring is the systematic and continuous collection, analysis and interpretation of sanitary/medical information relevant to public health.

The objectives of epidemiologic monitoring are:

- Follow-up of tendencies (estimate the impact of a disease or health problem through time; estimate dispersion of a disease, problem or incident; determination of risk factors);
- Localization of epidemics or cases (detection of epidemics/cases; prognosis of epidemics);
- Evaluation of public health management (evaluation of interventions; evaluation of public health strategies; follow-up of progress of objectives);
- Comprehension of health problems and their natural course.

These are types of epidemiologic monitoring subsystems:

- System of mandatory disease reporting (Fig. 11.1);
- System of illness observers in primary care (sentinel physicians);
- System of laboratory reporting;
- Syndromic surveillance;
- Networks (laboratories, early warning, monitoring of hospital infections).

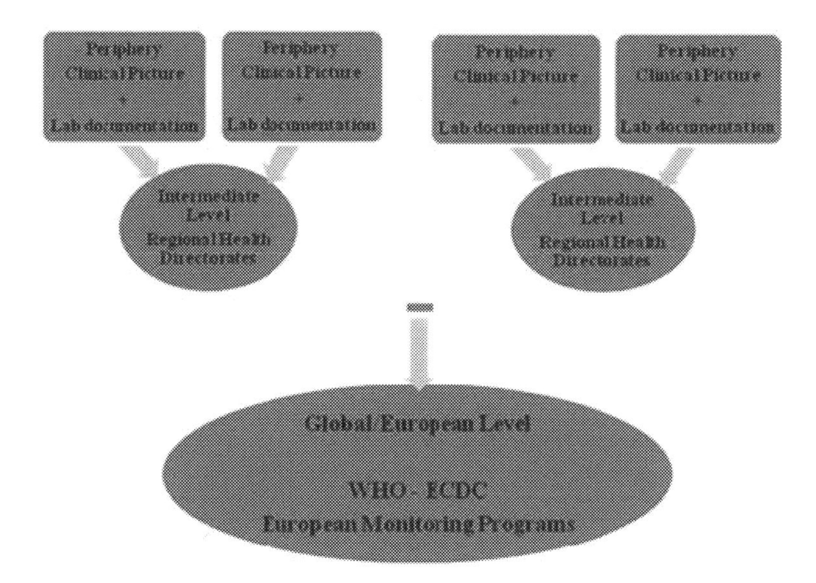

Fig. 11.1 Data flow during epidemiologic monitoring

11.4.2 Analysis of the Different Types of Epidemiologic Monitoring Systems

The system of mandatory reporting of diseases represents the basis of epidemiologic monitoring in most countries; usually it is supplemented by more specialized systems, networks or studies with specific objectives.

The objectives of this system are:

- Specific (for the system of mandatory reporting of diseases) – detection of sporadic cases; Detection of epidemic cases
- Generic (for every system of epidemiologic monitoring) – estimation of repercussions of illness through time; estimation of dissemination of illness; determination of risk factors; evaluation of interventions, evaluation of public health strategies, follow-up of progress of objectives.
- Diseases included in mandatory reporting:
  - Diseases belonging to a control or elimination programme;
  - Diseases for which direct preventive measures are required;
  - Diseases which can be identified in the event of an epidemic elevation at the local level;
  - Diseases for which the epidemiologic information is essential for the mapping of a long-term control policy.

Mandatory disease reporting systems intensified during the 2003–2004 period. During that time a complete revision of the 45 supervised diseases took place along with complete reformation of CDCP's databases aiming to reinforce a reliable system of mandatory reporting during the Olympic Games in Athens (2004). The Epidemiologic Monitoring and Intervention Division of CDCP was fully reformed to comply with the European Network of Epidemiologic Surveillance.

11.4.3 Categorization of Diseases of Mandatory Reporting

- Diseases of direct reporting (reporting immediately when explicit clinical suspicion exists) include: plague, anthrax, botulism, viral hemorrhagic fevers, smallpox, tularemia, Lassa virus, diphtheria, encephalitis from arthropod-borne viruses, rabies, cholera, and SARS.
- Diseases that are transmitted through the respiratory system or with droplets (reporting within 24 h following diagnosis) include: tuberculosis, legionellosis, meningitis of different types, and influenza (laboratory confirmed).
- Diseases that are prevented with vaccination (reporting within 24 h following diagnosis) include: tetanus/tetanus neonatal, whooping cough, measles, mumps, rubella, varicella (chickenpox) with complications, toxoplasmosis, and syphilis.
- Diseases that are transmitted through food, water or environmental sources, animal diseases, and viral hepatitis (reporting within 24 h following diagnosis) include: a large number of food-borne or water-borne diseases, typhoid fever, salmonellosis, shigellosis, infection with entero-haemorrhagic E. coli (EHEC), trichinellosis, brucellosis, listeria, Q fever, Echinococcus, leishmaniasis, leptospirosis, hepatitis A, hepatitis B (HBsAG (+) in infant of <12 months), and hepatitis C (confirmed Anti-HCV (+) first diagnosis).
- Diseases of special reporting and imported diseases (reporting within one week following diagnosis) include: AIDS, contagious spongiform encephalopathy (variant of CJD), poliomyelitis, and malaria.

11.4.4 Flow of Information

The reporting process can start from the clinical or laboratory doctor or the hospital's infectious diseases nurse but has to be sent immediately (by fax) to the Regional Health Directorates and CDCP.

The reporting form includes the following data:

- Full name;
- Date of birth or age;
- Residence/actual address;
- Connection with a similar case;
- Education;
- Nationality;
- Date of beginning of symptoms;
- Risk factors/precautions;

- Clinical characteristics;
- Laboratory results;
- Case classification.

After reporting, evaluation of the validity/completeness of the reported elements will follow along with a thorough investigation of the case that will lead to a systematic/rapid analysis and interpretation/export of the conclusions. Briefing of public health/sanitary/medical/nursing services will follow a complete evaluation of the system.

11.4.5 Legal Framework on Mandatory Reporting in Greece

1836: elementary mandatory reporting of diseases (Newspaper of Government, No. 83, 31/12/1836).

1911–1915: legislation on systematic mandatory reporting of diseases (cholera 1911, smallpox 1911, plague 1915).

1950: "Measures taken against infectious diseases justifying their reporting as mandatory", Art. 1: mandatory reporting of diseases (RD 7/9-11-1950).

1998: Essential improvement of mandatory reporting system (National Centre of Epidemiologic Surveillance and Intervention).

2003: "Organization and modernization of public health services and other provisions", Art. 8, Law 3172/6-8-2003: epidemiologic monitoring of pestiferous diseases is practiced and coordinated by CDCP.

2003: "Regulations applied for regional systems of health and providence", Art. 44, Law 3204/23-12-2003: CDCP – each private or public medical institution or individual doctor, operating legally, is obliged to inform CDCP of each case of pestiferous disease that comes to his/her attention.

Hellenic Personal Data Protection Authority:

- 1997: "Protection of individuals from the manipulation/exposure of data of personal character", Art. 7, Law 2472/1997: Exceptionally, it is allowed:
  - If it concerns subjects of health;
  - If it is executed by a health professional in duty of secrecy;
  - If it is essential for medical prevention.
- 2004: Authorization from "Hellenic Personal Data Protection Authority".

11.4.6 System of Illness Observers in the Primary Care Setting (Sentinel Physicians)

This system was set in operation in 1999 and revised in September 2004. It deals with common diseases with minor indications (usually). Its scope is to support the health system through data gathering and processing, to make a clear estimate of diachronic trends and detect a possible epidemic elevation in an area or region.

A large number of selected primary care doctors participate in this system/programme. These doctors are distributed all over the country in the following networks:

- Private doctors network (86 physicians);
- Regional health care centres/clinics (98 physicians);
- Social security institute health units network (44 physicians).

The diseases included in the system of illness observers at the first degree health care centres are: whooping cough, measles, mumps, rubella, varicella, influenza of infective etiology, respiratory infection with fever (>37.5 °C).

A weekly report is done of the number of cases and patients. The report is done according to the clinical findings and definitions.

11.4.7 Laboratory Reporting System

Laboratory reporting is an additional source of information. The objectives of this system are to provide health directorates a clear estimate of general tendencies over the years and provide them with the capability of detecting an epidemic elevation in the region.

Chosen laboratories with a suitable geographic distribution participate in the system/programme.

Prerequisites for the optimal function of the system include:

- Systematic weekly reporting;
- Sharing small amounts of information with constant flow from the laboratories;
- Sending cultures to specialized centres.

11.4.8 Syndromic Surveillance (Special Systems)

This system is activated in special conditions or when there is a specific objective. It applies to the reporting of predetermined clinical conditions ("syndromes") and not diagnosed diseases (e.g. "respiratory infection with fever" instead of "pneumonia from pneumococci").

Syndromic surveillance applies to the system of illness observers, early detection of epidemic elevations or individual incidents with public health importance (e.g. Olympic Games 2004) and in the case of a known epidemic (e.g. SARS).

Syndromes that are supervised with syndromic surveillance include:

- Respiratory infection;
- Hemorrhagic diarrhea;
- Gastroenteritis;
- Fever with rash;

- Meningitis (syndrome compatible with meningitis, encephalitis or unexplained acute encephalopathy/delirium);
- Hepatitis A (syndrome compatible with acute hepatitis);
- Syndrome compatible with botulism;
- Septic/unexplained shock;
- Unexplained death.

Other networks (laboratories, early warning, monitoring of hospital infections) and studies with specific objectives also exist. These are clinical-laboratory networks for special pathogens, such as hospital bio-pathology laboratories, reference laboratories, specialized laboratories, and special clinical units.

These networks focus on:

- Diseases of food origin (centres for Salmonella reporting);
- Contagious spongiform encephalopathy (centres for spongiform encephalopathy reporting);
- Poliomyelitis (centres for poliovirus reporting);
- Meningitis (centres for meningitis reporting);
- Legionellosis (centres for legionellosis reporting).

11.5 Military and Civilian agencies' Contribution in Preparedness and Response Against Natural or Deliberate Health Emergencies in Greece

All public sector services, in the case of a suspected or confirmed biological incident – deliberate or not – that needs to be treated, alert the Civil Protection Operations' Centre of GSCP.

GSCP then activates the Crisis Management Team (CMT) which consists of representatives from Police, Fire Service, First Aid National Center (FANC) [7], National Defence General Staff, Centre for Disease Control and Prevention (CDCP) and the GSCP itself.

GSCP's representative coordinates the functions of the CMT through telephone or video conference. After the thorough evaluation of the severity of the incident and the classification with different color codes if necessary, CMT will conduct a meeting at the GSCP building for better coordination of the operation.

When an initial estimation has been made, medical directorates in various/all regions of the country are informed and guidelines are issued. Medical directorates are obliged to report immediately to the GSCP about any laboratory result following citizens' examinations and inform the public according to the guidelines of GSCP.

Different missions are given to Police and Fire Service depending on the incident's nature.

If needed, National Defence General Staff contributes resources through its military hospitals, laboratories, mobile laboratories, medical personnel, services (mass vaccination) and equipment (direct supply of masks with filters against biological agents, personal protective suits, decontaminants, antidotes, drugs, mobile toilets, and decontamination facilities) or other supportive units (e.g. to clear or secure an area, for quick transportation or relocation of people, etc.).

In case of a CBRN agent release, Hellenic National Defence General Staff activates its Special Joint CBRN Company which has the capability to be airborne and deploy anywhere in Greece within 4 h (maximum), to conduct a CBRN search, survey, identification, sampling, decontamination, and provide specialized first aid. For bioterrorism agents, this company has the capability to operate portable biological detectors that can identify pathogens of special interest, such as those causing anthrax or plague, within 30 min (up to 28 biological samples can be processed simultaneously).

The Platoon was established after the 2004 Olympic Games by merging the two specialized units (one field unit operating in both hot and warm zones and one hospital-based unit deployed at the Army General Hospital of Athens) that were created and deployed during the Games in support of first responders.

References and Further Reading

1. Bailey KC (1994) Weapons of mass destruction: costs versus benefits. Manohar Publishers and Distributors, New Delhi
2. Center for Diseases Control and Prevention (CDCP). http://www.keelpno.gr
3. General Secretariat for Civil Protection (GSCP). http://www.gscp.gr
4. Ministerial Decision (MD) no. 3384/2006 "Supplement to the general plan for civil protection "XENOKRATES" with the specialized plan for the Management of Human Casualties"
5. Ministry of Citizen Protection. http://www.minocp.gov.gr
6. Ministry of Health and Social Solidarity. http://www.yyka.gov.gr
7. National First Aid Center (NFAC). http://www.ekab.gr

Chapter 12
Case Study – Israel

Adini Bruria, Manfred S. Green, and Daniel Laor

Abstract The risk of bioterrorism in Israel has been perceived in the last few decades as a very serious threat. Maintaining preparedness for both natural and human-made biological events poses a great challenge to the healthcare system. The Israeli model for emergency preparedness is based on five main components: (1) comprehensive contingency planning, (2) command of operations, (3) central control, (4) coordination and cooperation, and (5) capacity building of healthcare personnel. The response for all types of emergencies is based on the all-hazards approach. Three main legal frameworks facilitate effective management of the healthcare system during times of emergency, including the Public Health Ordinance (1940),

A. Bruria (✉)
Emergency and Disaster Management Division,
Ministry of Health, Tel Aviv, Israel

Department of Emergency Medicine, Faculty of Health Sciences,
Ben-Gurion University of the Negev, Beer-Sheva, Israel

PREPARED Research Center for Emergency Response Research,
Ben-Gurion University of the Negev, Beer-Sheva, Israel
e-mail: adini@netvision.net.il

M.S. Green
School of Public Health, University of Haifa, Haifa, Israel
e-mail: manfred.s.green@gmail.com

D. Laor
Emergency and Disaster Management Division,
Ministry of Health, Tel Aviv, Israel

PREPARED Research Center for Emergency Response Research,
Ben-Gurion University of the Negev, Beer-Sheva, Israel
e-mail: daniel@moh.health.gov.il

I. Hunger et al. (eds.), *Biopreparedness and Public Health: Exploring Synergies*,
NATO Science for Peace and Security Series A: Chemistry and Biology,
DOI 10.1007/978-94-007-5273-3_12,

the Civil Defense Law (1951) and the National Health Insurance Act (1995). These allow for great flexibility and wide authority of the health care leaders to manage responses to communicable diseases, pandemics and bioterror events.

12.1 Introduction

Funding emergency preparedness and response in Israel is provided by three main entities: (1) Ministry of Defense (responsible for procuring national stockpiles of personal protective gear, medications and vaccinations), (2) Ministry of Health (responsible for constructing vital infrastructure in the medical facilities and purchase of life-saving equipment to facilitate surge capacity), and (3) the medical institutions themselves (cover the costs for maintaining an ongoing readiness to respond to emergencies). The gradual and covert characteristics of a biological event necessitate operation of the following mechanisms: (1) ongoing surveillance systems, (2) expertise in epidemiological investigations, (3) isolation facilities, (4) shift of focus from acute-care hospitals to community health services, (5) protection of staff in order to elevate willingness to report to duty, and (6) provision of childcare centres outside medical facilities. A full collaboration between civilian and military systems is maintained in both preparedness and response phases of biological events. Senior military medical officers partner in formulating policies and implementing them during real events. National and regional exercises are initiated and conducted in the medical facilities, facilitated by the Home Front Command while logistic assistance and control and command of special operations, such as mass vaccinations, are provided by the Medical Corps or the Home Front Command. Maintaining readiness and preparedness for bioterrorism requires risk assessments to prioritize threats, development of policies and standard operating procedures, planning ahead, learning lessons from drills and biological events such as pandemics, and keeping a constant alert. Continuous ongoing readiness and preparedness enable the medical system to fulfill its purpose and save lives.

12.2 Public Health Threats

Biological agents do not recognize borders, therefore most countries in the Middle East share common threats to public health, in routine times as well as in emergencies. An example of this phenomenon is the measles outbreak that began in the Ramallah District of the Palestinian Authority in 1991 and spread to Israel a few weeks later [21]. Various types of zoonotic diseases have been identified in Israel such as the West Nile virus that caused outbreak of human disease since the 1950s [9]; the H5N1 outbreak in poultry in 2005–2006 [13]; and H1N1 pandemic influenza in 2009–2010. Additional zoonotic diseases include *Leishmania tropica* [20], *Bartonella spp.* [15] and brucellosis [18].

The broad geographic dispersal of pathogens is characteristic of the modern world and is similar in most countries. As such, Israel is susceptible to the same novel infectious disease threats [11] and non-infectious threats such as chemical and environmental threats or product contamination [5]. The risk of bioterrorism exists in Israel as it does in other parts of the world, though there is some debate as to the probability of its occurrence [8].

12.2.1 Perception of Bioterorrism as a Potential Threat

The risk of bioterrorism in Israel has been perceived since the 1990s as a very serious threat [6]. During the last decade, considerable resources have been devoted to the development and implementation of a national response plan [19].

12.2.2 Risk Assessment

Risk assessment is an ongoing process targeted to identify potential threats to the population's public health. The risk assessment process is designed to prevent, mitigate, and manage potential emergency scenarios [17]. In Israel, the process of risk assessment regarding biological events (both natural and man-made) involves three main entities: the Ministry of Defense that focuses mainly on threats of bioterrorism; the Ministry of Health (MoH) that prepares for all types of events, including natural events, intentional or unintended risks (such as laboratory or research accidents), and designated research centres. The result of this process is the determination of the probability and potential consequences of the biological event and, based on this information, development of a response plan. The mechanism for conducting risk assessment is described in Fig. 12.1 [1].

12.2.3 Classification into Families – Viral, Bacterial, Toxins, Pandemics

There are numerous agents that pose a biological threat on the public health. Developing a designated response to each type of threat can be both confusing and non-productive to the healthcare personnel. Therefore, a generic response model characterizes the preparedness to manage these potential events. Nevertheless, as there are specific differences between the agents, the preparedness is designed to suit four main families as follows [16]:

- Viral agents such as viral encephalitides, viral hemorrhagic fevers, and smallpox.
- Toxins such as aflatoxin, botulinum, and ricin.
- Bacterial diseases such as anthrax, brucellosis, plague, Q fever, and tularemia.
- Pandemic influenza resulting from antigenic shift such as H5N1 and H1N1.

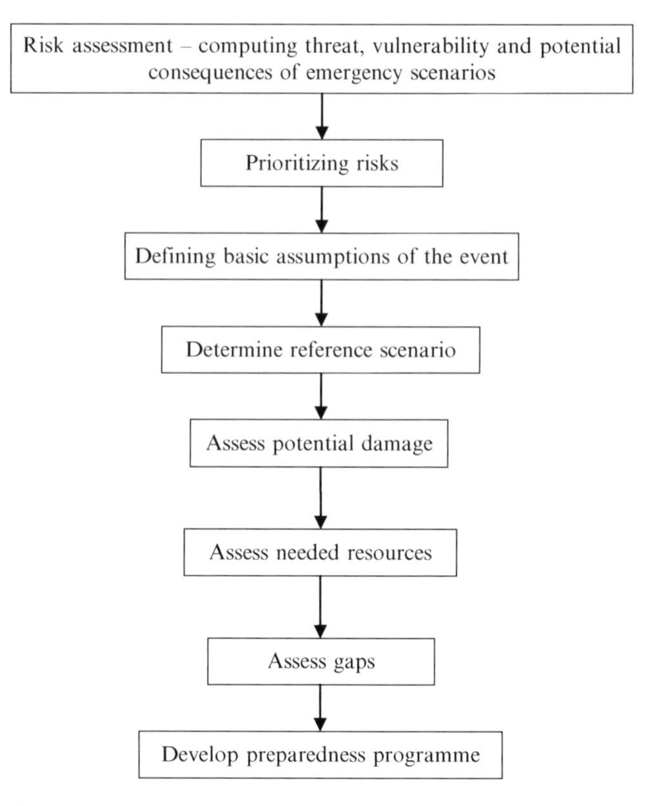

Fig. 12.1 Risk assessment process in Israel

12.3 Preparedness and response to health emergencies in Israel

The emergency preparedness response plan is based on a 5 C model composed of: (1) comprehensive contingency planning, (2) command of operations, (3) central control, (4) coordination and cooperation, and (5) capacity building of healthcare personnel [1–3].

12.3.1 Comprehensive Contingency Planning

The response model for all types of emergencies is based on the all-hazards approach as there are common components of emergency management regardless of the specific type of scenario [22]. Preparedness for a multi-casualty incident serves as the basis for the preparedness and needed modifications are implemented, such as personal protection gear and decontamination capabilities for toxicological or chemical events and vaccinations or anti-viral medications for a biological event. The aim is to create mechanisms for a generic universal response to the various threats.

The doctrines are developed nationally, by special committees and task forces that are nominated by the MoH. They are then disseminated to the medical organizations that adapt them into institutional standard operating procedures (SOPs), based on their resources and infrastructure. The institutional plans must be reviewed and approved by the MoH or the Home Front Command (authorized for this activity by the MoH).

Designated equipment (such as personal protective gear or life saving equipment) and pharmaceuticals (such as antibiotics for anthrax) required to treat casualties and patients that are admitted to the medical facilities during emergencies, are procured by the MoH. At times, these are produced locally by the MoH, such as the vaccines or Vaccinia Immune Globulin (VIG) for smallpox. Some of the equipment is stored in national warehouses spread across several geographic locations and the remainder is distributed to the medical facilities to ensure their immediate availability for deployment in times of need.

Relevant infrastructure, such as decontamination facilities or isolation facilities, is installed in the medical facilities by the MoH, regardless of the ownership of these institutions (governmental, Health Maintenance Organization (HMO), non-governmental organizations (NGOs), or private facilities).

12.3.2 Command of Operations

The overall responsibility for preparing and managing a bioterror event in Israel is under the jurisdiction of the Ministry of Defense. The National Emergency Management Agency (NEMA) is the highest authority that functions as the overall coordinator and directs operation of the various governmental ministries. The healthcare system is managed by the Supreme Health Authority (SHA) which is the highest authority operated by the MoH (see Fig. 12.2). It is headed by the director-general of the MoH and the other members include the director-general of the largest Health Maintenance Organization (HMO) and the Surgeon-General of the Medical Corps in the Israeli Defense Force (IDF). In the meetings of this authority, representatives participate from all relevant agencies including the three additional HMOs, the emergency medicine services, the Home Front Command, and NEMA. The SHA convenes regularly during routine times to develop operational doctrines for all healthcare institutions and to follow-up their effective implementation. During a biological event, such as the last A/H1N1 influenza pandemic, it convenes twice a day, usually utilizing teleconference channels.

In order to deploy the emergency response and monitor its implementation, the SHA conducts professional forums during prolonged events (conflicts or biological events) that serve as the basis for information flow and direct communication. Daily teleconferences are also conducted with directors of acute-care hospitals as well as primary care institutions including the directors of all four HMOs and health district officers.

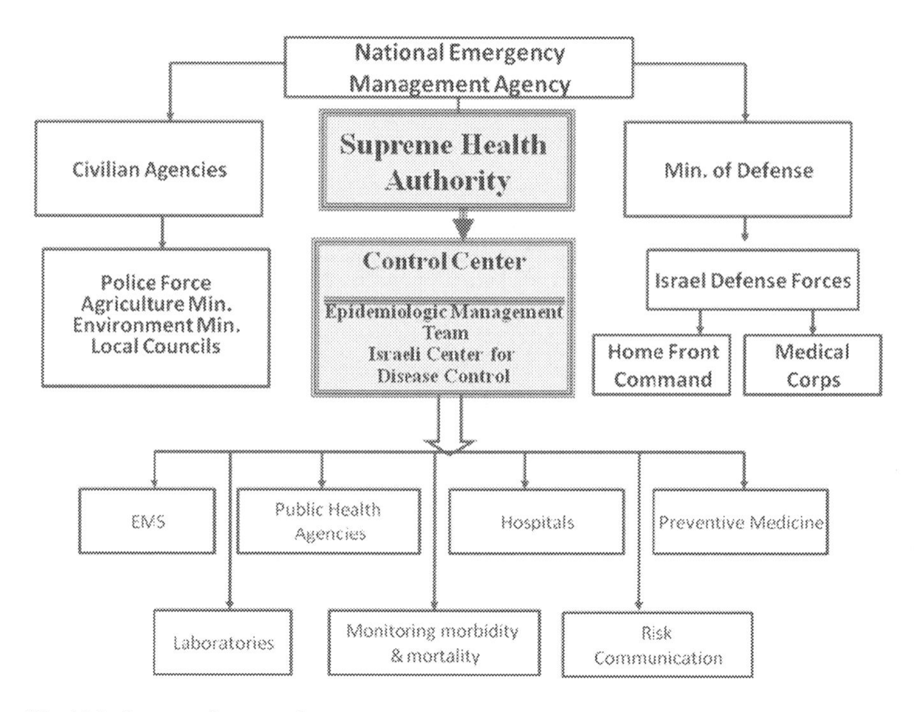

Fig. 12.2 Structure for managing an event

12.3.3 Central Control of Emergency Readiness and Preparedness

Maintaining readiness to respond to emergencies requires an ongoing evaluation of preparedness. Such evaluation facilitates identification of strengths and weaknesses and encourages continuous improvement of emergency preparedness. The evaluation is based on a structured tool that includes approximately 1,000 measurable and objective parameters, amongst them 300 parameters that measure readiness for biological events. These evaluations are conducted once every 2 years in all acute-care hospitals and once every 3 years in the primary care institutions. The evaluators consist of employees from the MoH and the Home Front Command that are experts in the areas evaluated. A follow-up is conducted to ensure implementation of findings presented in the evaluation.

Ongoing capabilities of the medical institutions are monitored based on three information systems: (1) on-line admission data (ATD systems) that continually transmit information regarding utilization of hospital beds, including admittance and discharge of patients in the emergency departments, (2) web-based daily reports on critical services (such as the number of ventilated patients), and (3) a geographic information system (GIS) that enables a continuous surveillance to manage communicable diseases and bioterror events. The GIS maps the medical institutions and facilitates recognition of available medical services and monitoring spread of infectious diseases.

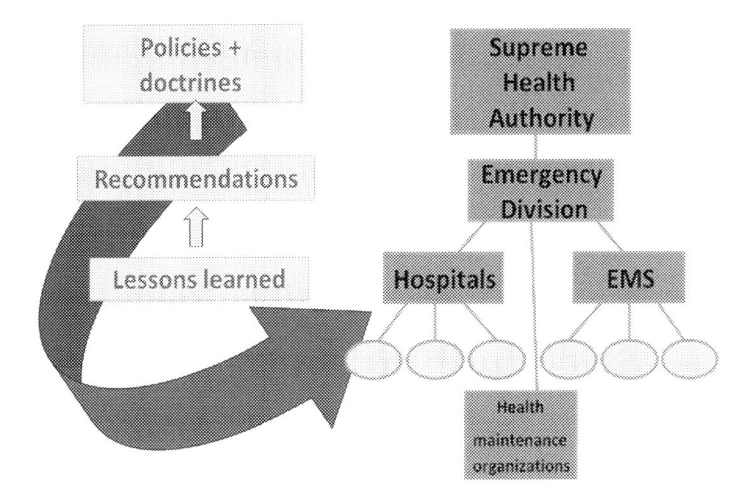

Fig. 12.3 Conduct of an After Action Review

A crucial component of the central control is the conduct of an After Action Review (AAR) following every type of emergency, such as a mass casualty incident (MCI), a toxicological event, or the occurrence of the H1N1 influenza pandemic. The AAR is conducted in three levels; initially in the organizational level (hospital, HMO or emergency medical service); secondly in the regional level headed and chaired by the Emergency & disaster management division of the MoH and finally in the level of the Supreme Health Authority (see Fig. 12.3). A structured AAR tool is utilized to facilitate the process of identifying and learning lessons.

An additional important component is the dictated level of surge capacity that the acute care hospitals have to maintain in order to manage an immediate response to an emergency scenario. The MoH dictates three levels of surge that each hospital is required to prepare for: (1) expansion of surge capacity for immediate MCIs at an extent of 20% of the total routine bed capacity, (2) expansion of surge capacity for prolonged emergencies such as conflicts with neighboring countries, at an extent of between 40 and 60% of routine bed capacity, and (3) expansion of surge capacity for biological events at an extent of 60% of routine bed capacity. In order to effectively prepare for these expansions, the MoH provides the hospitals with the necessary equipment and infrastructure.

12.3.4 *Coordination and Cooperation Among the Various Emergency Agencies*

Coordination and cooperation among the various emergency agencies is achieved by the following main components: (1) development of joint doctrines so that common terminology is utilized by the different agencies and all teams can be easily acquainted with the responsibilities and activities of interface forces, (2) joint communication channels and mechanisms installed to facilitate sharing of information and relay relevant data during emergencies, (3) joint drills and exercises that are conducted annually in which representatives from the various medical institutions such as hospitals, primary care facilities, health districts, ministerial bodies etc. participate, and (4) liaison officers who are deployed upon an occurrence of an emergency to ensure flow of information and facilitate effective utilization of resources.

12.3.5 Capacity Building

National and regional training programmes are initiated by the MoH in order to ensure knowledge and capabilities of the healthcare personnel. Advanced training materials such as video films, computerized software and training kits are produced on a national level and disseminated to the various healthcare institutions to be utilized in conducting annual training programmes. Representatives from all the healthcare agencies are trained by the MoH and then function in their institutions as "nucleus knowledge groups" in charge of training relevant personnel. The development and implementation of training programmes are evaluated by the MoH as part of the evaluations that are conducted to assess the level of emergency preparedness. Regional simulation exercises are held in which representatives from the different institutions participate. These enhance multidisciplinary communication and coordination between intra and inter sectors. A compulsory exercise programme is dictated by the Supreme Health Authority and the performance levels are measured and assessed, as well as follow-up of implementing lessons learned.

12.4 Legal Frameworks

Israel has developed a legal framework to ensure a response to emergencies [4]. Three main legal frameworks facilitate effective management of the healthcare system during times of emergency, the Public Health Ordinance (1940), the Civil Defense Law (1951), and the National Health Insurance Act (1995).

12.4.1 The Public Health Ordinance

The Public Health Ordinance was enacted when Israel was under the British mandate and was adopted by the Israeli government upon the creation of the State in 1948. This law provides the MoH with an extensive tool to respond to public health threats, focusing on communicable diseases. Under this law, the Director-General of the MoH is authorized to compel any person, healthcare employee or medical institution to take any action deemed necessary in order to prevent, mitigate or limit consequences of a biological event. Among other actions, the Director-General can direct healthcare providers to conduct house calls, supply all medical and public health services, bury the dead, detain for medical inspection travelers from infected areas, procure land or buildings to accommodate detained population, and forbid exit from infected area. These extensive authorities provide the MoH administration with powerful tools to control epidemics and pandemics.

12.4.2 The Civil Defense Law

The Civil Defense Law enables the Home Front Command to direct operations of the Emergency Medical Services (EMS) and HMOs during times of emergencies (wartime or during conflicts), to ensure their continued operation. Based on this law, employees in crucial services can be compelled to report to work.

12.4.3 The National Health Insurance Act

The National Health Insurance Act ensures the rights of the population to receive medical services in times of emergencies as well as in routine times. It also commits the HMOs to ensure availability and accessibility of medical services to the population, both in routine times and in emergencies.

12.5 Funding Emergency Preparedness and Response

Attaining sufficient funding to maintain a continuous preparedness to emergencies proves to be a challenge in most countries; therefore, cost-sharing between the various stakeholders is highly recommended [14]. Funding of emergency preparedness and response in Israel is provided by three main entities: Ministry of Defense, Ministry of Health, and the institutions themselves. National stockpiles of personal protective gear, medications, and vaccinations are procured by the Ministry of Defense which also funds extensive research designated to improving security measures and protection of the population and the first responders. Construction of vital infrastructure in medical facilities such as decontamination sites, permanent or mobile isolation rooms, etc. is funded by the MoH, along with the purchase of life-saving medical equipment, equipment required to facilitate surge capacity of hospitals, or other vital products such as appliances for expansion of operating rooms. The MoH also finances development of training materials and direct costs of drills and exercises, such as transportation of mock casualties.

The costs for maintaining an ongoing readiness to respond to emergencies are covered by each institution including funding of the development of institutional SOPs, conduct of training and drills (loss of income which is incurred when some of the services are withheld during the time of the exercise, overtime etc.), and renewal of equipment that was allocated by the MoH. The medical institutions are not reimbursed for costs required for ensuring emergency preparedness as this is considered part of their obligation to provide high level medical care to the population, in both routine and emergency times.

12.6 Differences in Preparedness and Response to a Bioterrorism Event in Relation to Other Health Emergencies

Emergency response systems are often designed to prepare for and respond to short-term incidents rather than emergencies that necessitate ongoing response mechanisms [7]. A biological event requires continuous mechanisms for both the preparedness and response phases.

12.6.1 Need to Operation Ongoing Surveillance Systems

Most types of emergencies, such as multi-casualty events, mass toxicological events, natural disasters, or man-made conflicts, are overt and their occurrence is immediately recognized. A biological event is very different and recognition of its occurrence poses a greater challenge. The time from occurrence to development of casualties is very rapid in most types of emergencies (caused immediately by the event) while it is much more gradual in a biological event (patients may present signs and symptoms days after exposure). The extent of influence of the emergency might also vary between biological and other types of emergencies. As in most types of emergency scenarios, the affected population will consist of those that were directly present at the time of occurrence, while biological agents may cause communicable diseases and pandemics and can affect a much larger spread of the population.

In order to prepare an effective response to the unique characteristics of biological events (both natural and man-made), there is a need to develop and sustain an ongoing surveillance system. The goal is to monitor morbidity and mortality of the population along with additional relevant data, to facilitate early rapid detection and identification of such an event. While it is recognized that the surveillance system itself will, most probably, not be the mechanism that will present the initial alert that an exceptional event has occurred (clinicians are believed to be the best sentinels), it is still a vital tool to assist in the management of such an event.

12.6.2 Epidemiological Investigations

Upon recognition that a biological event has occurred, in most cases there will still be a need to identify the cause of the event, its characteristics and accordingly to determine the case definition. The mechanism to achieve these goals is through epidemiological investigations. This process must include search of relevant information, interview of sources, sharing of data, and analysis of findings as well as advanced laboratory capacities to detect and identify pathogens. The epidemiological investigation provides the basis for decision and policy makers in directing operations and managing the response.

12.6.3 Isolation Facilities

In view of the potential threat of mass infections and communicable diseases, there is a need to provide isolation facilities to be utilized in biological events. While this element is not needed in most types of emergencies, in biological events it is a vital component of the response model. Isolated conditions can be provided by installing permanent or temporary isolation rooms to which the patients suffering from communicable diseases will be confined. Towards this, the MoH purchased mobile isolation rooms that will be distributed to medical facilities during pandemics or other outbreaks of communicable diseases. An alternate mode of operation is isolation of biological patients from other types of patients by utilizing designated medical facilities which will treat solely the biological patients. Nevertheless, this type of operation may prove to be both complicated and resource-consuming.

12.6.4 Shift of Focus from Acute-Care Hospitals to Community Health Services

The response model for most types of emergencies is based on operation of pre-hospital EMS services and acute-care hospitals. The primary care institutions are usually not involved in the provision of emergency services to casualties and only serve to provide post-hospital care to discharged patients. In a biological event, there is a distinct shift of focus and primary care institutions, HMOs and health districts services are expected to carry the highest burden. Hospitals are designated to treat only severely ill patients, especially those needing ventilation and extensive medical support, while light or moderately ill patients are directed to receive medical attention provided in the community.

Medical services in the community are provided by one of the following mechanisms:

- Medical clinics operated by the four HMOs. These medical services can be provided in either institutional clinics consisting of several physicians, nurses, and at times pharmacy services, or in individual clinics operated by private physicians employed by the HMOs.
- Exposure Centres utilized specifically for biological events. These centres consist of medical personnel, civilian and military, designated to provide vaccinations and medications to patients based on case definitions defined by public health officials from the MoH.

12.6.5 Willingness to Report to Duty – Preparedness to Provide Protective Measures

Healthcare providers are known for their commitment to their place of work and to their obligation to provide life-saving services to the needy. As part of this obligation, in the different emergency scenarios that Israel has had to contend with, there was never a shortage of staff resulting from refusal to report to duty; the opposite was more characteristic – there was a surplus of employees that rushed to their medical facilities, eager to contribute to the care of patients and casualties. Nevertheless, when preparing for a biological event, the possibility of staff failure to report to work caused by fear of becoming ill should be considered by healthcare management. Fear of infection to employees or risk to their families must be addressed by provision of information regarding risks and counter-measures, availability of protective measures such as personal protective gear or preventive medications (if available), and conditions to ensure safety of family members.

12.6.6 Operating Childcare Centres Outside the Medical Facilities

As a result of lessons learned from various types of disasters, childcare centres are immediately operated within all acute-care hospitals upon an occurrence of a prolonged emergency. This measure facilitates willingness of healthcare employees to report to work during various emergency scenarios. While it is crucial to provide such services also in biological events, it does not seem appropriate to locate them at the hospitals themselves, considering the added risk of infection. Therefore, in this type of event, there is a need to provide an alternate solution to childcare of healthcare employees. Deploying childcare centres in the community, in cooperation with local councils and education institutions, is deemed necessary, along with arrangement of accessible transportation to both employees and their children.

12.7 Role of the Military in Preparedness and Response to Health Emergencies

In a small country such as Israel, optimal utilization of resources in response to emergencies can only be achieved if full collaboration between the civilian and military systems is maintained. Coordination between these two systems can easily be identified in both preparedness and response phases of biological events. The relationship consists of a civilian-defence partnership characterized by a distinct structure of interface between governmental, military, and civilian agencies [12].

12.7.1 Policy Making

Senior military medical officers are members of the Supreme Health Authority and are therefore part of the mechanism for formulating policies to manage emergencies and implementing them in the healthcare system. The Surgeon General of the IDF is a full member of this Authority and the Chief Medical Officer of the Home Front Command participates in the discussions and is frequently responsible for implementing its decisions. Military representatives are significant partners in defining policies for emergency response and for their operation during emergency events. Military personnel serve as members in all the advisory committees including in the Epidemic Management Team (EMT) designated to recommend lines of actions in natural and man-made biological events.

12.7.2 Training and Exercises

Ensuring integration of knowledge among healthcare personnel and its sustainability over time necessitates an ongoing programme for training and exercises. This is a complex challenge as there is a need to include in these activities multi-disciplinary representatives from numerous institutions such as the HMOs, health districts, acute-care hospitals, and administration officials from the MoH, as well as interface agencies such as the Ministry of Defense, agriculture authorities, and others. Each year several exercises are conducted including at least one extensive regional exercise. The Home Front Command fully collaborates with the MoH to initiate and conduct these exercises. In order to assist in the preparation of such training and exercise programmes, the Home Front Command has established two branches – a hospitalization branch and a community branch – designated to assist the medical institutions to prepare for emergencies. Military personnel from these two branches operate in complete coordination of the MoH and serve as an auxiliary resource to achieve emergency preparedness and response.

12.7.3 Logistical Assistance and Control and Command of Special Operations

Many actions required in the response to biological events entail complex logistical support. For example, in an emergence of smallpox, the national policy dictates massive vaccination of the population within four days [10]. The military system is the only practical means that can effectively implement this line of action. Therefore, the IDF and especially the Home Front Command are actively involved in development of response models and their implementation in the occurrence of a real event. Such involvements encompass the following: (1) Home Front Command is the authorized entity responsible for deployment, control and command of Exposure Centres planned to provide mass vaccinations or medications following a biological event; (2) Home Front Command is the leader and executor of the plan for rapid vaccination of the nation's population following an outbreak of smallpox; and (3) the military allocates soldiers to assist in operating day-care centres for children of healthcare providers during emergencies so as to facilitate their reporting to their place of work.

12.8 Conclusions

The Israeli model for emergency preparedness is based on five main components: comprehensive contingency planning; command of operations; central control; coordination and cooperation between emergency agencies; and capacity building. Maintaining readiness and preparedness for bioterrorism requires risk assessments in order to prioritize threats, development of policies and standard operating procedures, planning ahead, learning lessons from drills and biological events such as pandemics, and keeping a constant alert. Continuous ongoing readiness and preparedness enable the medical system to fulfill its purpose and save lives.

References

1. Adini B (2009) Hospital organization for conventional mass casualty incidents. In: Shapira S, Falk O (eds) Best practices for medical management of terror incidents. Robert Wood Johnson University Hospital, New Brunswick, NJ, p 187–222
2. Adini B, Goldberg A, Laor D, Cohen R, Zadok R, Bar-Dayan Y (2006) Assessing levels of hospital emergency preparedness. Prehosp Disaster Med 21(6):451–457
3. Adini B, Laor D, Cohen R, Israeli A (2010) The five commandments to preparedness of the Israeli healthcare system to emergencies. Harefuah 149(7):445–450
4. Barnett DJ, Balicer RD, Lucey DR, Everly GS Jr, Omer SB et al (2005) A systematic analytic approach to pandemic influenza preparedness planning. PLoS Med 2(12):e359
5. EpiSouth Project (2010) Epidemic intelligence and cross-border in the mediterranean countries and balkans. http://www.episouth.org/outputs/wp6/3_EpiSouth%20Strategic% 20document %20on%20Cross-Border%20Ep%20Int%20Rev%20luglio%202010.pdf

6. Friedman D, Rager-Zisman B, Bibi E, Keynan A (2010) The bioterrorism threat and dual-use biotechnological research: an Israeli perspective. Sci Eng Ethics 16(1):85–97
7. Gerber BJ, Robinson SE (2009) Local government performance and the challenges of regional preparedness for disasters. Public Perform Manag Rev 32(3):345–371
8. Green MS, Zenilaman J, Cohen D, Wiser I, Balicer RD (2007) Risk assessment and risk communication strategies in bioterrorism preparedness. Springer, Dordrecht
9. Gulcer DJ (2002) The global emergenci/resurgence of Arboviral diseased as public health problems. Arch Med Res 33:330–342
10. Huerta M, Balicer RD, Levnethal A (2003) SWOT analysis: strengths, weaknesses, opportunities and threats of the Israeli smallpox revaccination program. IMAG 5:42–46
11. Kimball AM, Moore M, French HM, Arima Y, Ungchusak K, Wibulpolprasert S et al (2008) Regional infectious disease surveillance networks and their potential to facilitate the implementation of the International Health Regulations. Med Clin N Am 92:1459–1471
12. Kohn S, Barnett DJ, Leventhal A, Reznikovich S, Oren M, Laor D, Grotto I, Balicer RD (2010) Pandemic influenza preparedness and response in Israel: a unique model of civilian-defense collaboration. J Public Health Policy 31:256–269
13. Leventhal A, Ramlawi A, Belbiesi A (2006) Regional collaboration in the Middle East to deal with H5N1 avian flu. BMJ 333(7573):856–858
14. MacManus SA, Caruson K (2008) Financing homeland security and emergency preparedness: use of inter-local cost-sharing. Public Budg Finance 28(2):48–68
15. Morick D, Baneth G, Avidor B, Kosoy MY, Mumcuoglu KY, Mintz D, Eyal O, Goethe R, Mietze A, Shpigel N, Harrus S (2009) Detection of *Bartonella* spp. In wild rodents in Israel using HRM real-time PCR. Vet Microbiol 139(3–4):293–297
16. Oren M (2009) Biological agents and terror medicine. In: Shapira SC, Hammond JS, Cole LA (eds) Essential in terror medicine. Springer, New York
17. Pelfrey WV (2005) The cycle of preparedness: establishing a framework to prepare for terrorist threats. J Homel Secur Emerg Manage 2(1):5
18. Sakran W, Chazan B, Koren A (2006) Brucellosis: clinical presentation, diagnosis, complications and therapeutic options. Harefuah 145(11):836–840, 860
19. Shapira SC, Oren M (2006) Ethical issues of bioterror. Stud Confl Terror 29(5):395–401
20. Talmi-Frank D, Kedem-Vaanunu N, King R, Bar-Gal GK, Edery N, Jaffe CL, Baneth G (2010) *Leishmania tropica* infection in golden jackals and red foxes. Israel Emerg Infect Dis 16(12):1973–1975
21. Tulchinsky TH, Belmaker I, Raabi S, Acker C, Arbeli Y, Lobel R, Abed Y, Toubassi N, Goldberg E, Slater PE (1992–1993) Measles during the Gulf War: a public health threat in Israel, the West Bank, and Gaza. Public Health Rev 20(3–4):285–296
22. Levy L, Rokusek C, Bragg SM, Howell J (2009) Interdisciplinary approach to all-hazards preparedness: are you ready? How do we know? J Public Health Manag Pract 15(2):S8–S12

Chapter 13
Case Study – Italy

Francesco Urbano and Maria Rita Gismondo

Abstract After the peak of interest in 2001, the threat of bioterrorism is now considered just one of the diverse risks Italy's society faces endangering public health. Without major investments, the effort has been to integrate existing resources, to implement tight links among national and supranational agencies and to make plans for their most efficient involvement in case of need. The mainstay for the response to a biological attack is represented by the public health system, entrusted to Italy's national health service, centrally coordinated but put into action by the Regions. The emerging threat of emerging infectious diseases and of bioterrorism has shown the need for a change in the education curricula of sanitary professions and for specific training of first line operators. Specific courses have been activated by universities and other bodies, but attendance has been limited by the lack of ad hoc funds.

13.1 Background

In the 150 years as a unitary state, Italy has always devoted much attention to its public health, starting with the Crispi-Pagliani law of 1888 which collated the several previous sanitary systems into a single one, centrally controlled and articulated in over 90 provincial medical offices and laboratories, and sanitary officers in the over 8,000 townships, with consistent public health structures in the large cities.

F. Urbano (✉)
Italian Army Logistic Branch, Medical Department, Rome, Italy
e-mail: francesco.urbano@esercito.difesa.it

M.R. Gismondo
Clinical Microbiology Laboratory, Faculty of Medicine and Surgery,
"Luigi Sacco" University Hospital, Milan, Italy
e-mail: mariarita.gismondo@unimi.it

I. Hunger et al. (eds.), *Biopreparedness and Public Health: Exploring Synergies*,
NATO Science for Peace and Security Series A: Chemistry and Biology,
DOI 10.1007/978-94-007-5273-3_13,

The fascist regime reordered the system in 1934, and implemented large programmes against tuberculosis and malaria. Several health care systems were activated for various working groups, and were eventually unified into the INAM (*Istituto Nazionale di Assicurazione contro le Malattie* – National Institute for Health Care Insurance).

After the war, with the advent of the Republic, its Constitution, Article 32, stated health to be a fundamental right of the individual and interest of the community [4]. In 1978, the previous health insurance system was abolished and the SSN (*Servizio Sanitario Nazionale* – National Health Service) was established on the model of the British NHS.

Again implementing the Constitution, in 1970 the autonomy of the 20 Regions had been recognized, and since 1980 they were charged with the management of health in their territories, in the frame of national sanitary programmes decided centrally by the health minister, with the assistance of various technical bodies, like the ISS (*Istituto Superiore di Sanità* – Superior Health Institute). Each Region has legislative power to implement the SSN in its territory, and provides health care through a number of hospitals, USL (*Unità Sanitarie Locali* – Local Sanitary Units) or ASL (*Aziende Sanitarie Locali* – Local Sanitary Enterprises). The SSN employs over 600,000 persons, including about 100,000 MDs and 260,000 nurses [24].

Presently the SSN is characterized by universality; it is funded by the general fiscality and it takes care both of clinical and preventive medicine. There are great efficiency gaps between Regions [18], and – although plagued by corruption, cronyism, and nepotism – Italy's SSN ranks among the best, as judged by WHO, and Italy's health profile is above regional and global averages [36].

13.2 Public Health in Italy

ASLs are responsible for the use of allotted resources in all aspects of health care; so they are also in charge of protecting and promoting public health; each has a section or department of preventive medicine that deals with hygiene and public health: epidemiology, health promotion and education, food control, veterinary surveillance, and environment protection.

Other agencies cooperate in the protection of public health, either at the regional level, like the ARPAs (*Agenzie Regionali di Protezione Ambientale* – Regional Environment Protection Agencies) or supra-regional, like the 10 IZPSs (*Istituti Zooprofilattici Sperimentali* – Experimental Zoo Prophylactic Institutes).

13.3 Coping with Emergencies

Perhaps more than other countries, Italy has suffered from a wide range of catastrophes, both natural – earthquakes, eruptions, floods (Polesine 1951; Florence 1966), landslides – and man-induced – wars, industrial disasters (Seveso 1976), railroad explosions (Viareggio 2009), terrorist massacres (Piazza Fontana 1969; Fiumicino

1973, 1985; Bologna 1980), forest fires, and epidemics. Through the centuries, the latter, especially the plague pandemics, have had an essential role in shaping the public health response that has been the basis for Italy's modern public health system, and a model elsewhere in Europe and the world [1, 5]. Of the former, the earlier ones have been met by improvisation; in time, they have driven the establishment of the present system to cope with all kinds of emergencies, mainly based on Civil Defence (*Difesa Civile* – DC), and Civil Protection (*Protezione Civile* – PC).

13.3.1 The Role of the Military

Italy used to have a compulsory military draft; the Army was a vast organization, diffuse across the territory and well structured; for decades it has been the mainstay of the response to all kinds of emergencies, with the obvious limits set by the lack of specific training [20].

In time, military service has become a specialized profession [13]. The Army has reduced its manpower and dismantled many of its territorial structures. Generally speaking, in the event of a disaster the role of the military has become subsidiary to that of the organizations whose mission is the defence and protection of the civilians. However, the specific threat posed by biological agents (and chemical or nuclear weapons) dictates that the military apparatus be ready to face it, so it maintains specialized units for NBC (nuclear, biological, chemical) defence, and a national centre for research and specific training, which is done at the Nubich grounds, near Rieti. The centre runs courses for the personnel of all the armed forces, the national and local police corps, the Italian Red Cross, the firemen, the SSN, and the railway and port authorities. The centre, which participates in international working groups, develops policies, procedures, and guidelines for the integrated response to NBCR emergencies. Although subsidiary, the role of the Army remains essential, on account of its logistics and the capacity to mobilize its manpower, including its specialized medical and engineer corps (Fig. 13.1). One particular unit, the 7th Regiment "Cremona", is fully dedicated to NBC defence; the regiment has specialized units for the delimitation of the affected area and for the decontamination of people and materials. Regarding the biological hazards, it is equipped with a mobile laboratory capable of molecular detection of biological agents, isolator tents, and ambulances.

A limited capacity for the safe aerial transport of highly contagious patients is guaranteed by the Air Force, with a number of aircraft transit isolators which, along with specially trained and equipped teams, have been used for civilian missions on several occasions.

13.3.2 Civil Defence (DC)

The notion of DC has changed in time and it has given rise to a variety of models. At present, in Italy, DC is conceived as a hierarchy of diverse structures which are

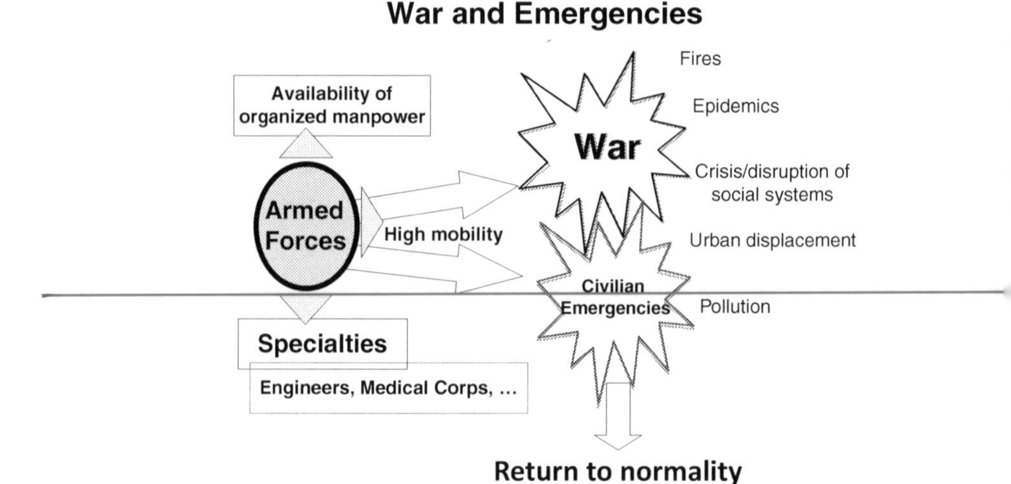

Fig. 13.1 The asset of the armed forces, conceived to face war, remains essential for the integrated response to all kinds of civilian emergencies. (Modified from [19])

coordinated to respond to intentional threats, including bioterrorism, which endanger the population. National (secret) intelligence services, in collaboration with the ones of other countries or organizations, should assess the risks of such threats.

The chain of command for DC has vertex structures at ministerial level, and provincial prefects who coordinate the efforts of municipal entities. Personnel and facilities may be drawn from the SSN, the PC structures, the military apparatus, the Red Cross, and volunteer NGOs. DC can activate emergency operational rooms at various levels and it may emanate and enforce regulations.

13.3.3 Civil Protection (PC)

The Law 225/1992 (24 February 1992) [17] has established a national department, at the highest ministerial level, with the mission to foresee, prevent, and manage extraordinary events that might endanger the population; Italy's PC is not directly aimed to face bioterrorism, but its structures may be called upon by the DC in order to activate an integrated response.

The organization of PC is diffuse on the territory, and it can rely on over 300,000 variously trained volunteers and on all the facilities available to public institutions. PC follows the so called "Augustus method", which formalizes the steps to be taken to the various ends of the mission. In particular, it links the various functions, in order to define the scenarios and to answer the questions "Who does what, where and when?" [10].

13.4 Biological Warfare

The idea that biological agents can be used as weapons dates back to pre-history [32]. In modern times several states have invested a lot for the study and development of biological weapons. There have been international agreements to ban them, which have not deterred some states, notably Japan, to use them, and others, notably the two superpowers, to prepare huge stockpiles of deadly, "weaponized" biological agents.

Italy had adhered to the Geneva Protocol of 1925, prohibiting the use in war of chemical or bacteriological methods of warfare. At the time, and until World War II, some experts were engaged in literature searches on the matter of the potential use of biological agents, and a limited amount of research was done on it. Contrary to a recent libel asserting a heavy involvement of the fascist regime in biological warfare [7], it is proven by documents from the British National Archives that the allies had investigated Italy's activities in the field and concluded that they were very limited in scope, lightly financed, and naively conducted [3].

Rather than an active actor, Italy appears to have been the victim of an insidious kind of biological warfare, the attack by the Germans to the reclamation system of marshy lands in the Pontine area, with the introduction of salty waters to favour the breeding of *Anopheles labranchiae*. There followed an upsurge of malaria cases, which lasted for years after the end of the war [28].

13.5 Bioterrorism

Worldwide, the concept of bioterrorism is recent, as it only emerged in the 1990s of the past century. A PubMed search for the word finds nothing until 1996, when a paper was published in JAMA [31]. An editorial of 1997 recognized the unpreparedness of society to face bioterrorism, and pleaded for more attention to the threat [35], while the six papers of 1998 stressed its relevance to public health. Figure 13.2 shows how the number of papers on bioterrorism rose at first slowly, and then peaked on account of the anthrax mailings following the Twin Tower attack of 11 September 2001.

In fact, the surge of scientific interest on bioterrorism was an immediate consequence of the new geopolitical asset of the world, with the end of the superpower bipolar influence, which had been based on atomic deterrence. Biological agents were thus considered to be attractive by "rogue states" and by non-governmental groups, on account of their favourable cost/effects ratios, which allowed their economic development as weapons of mass destruction or their use as a frightening means of terrorism, capable, with a modest effort, of disrupting entire societies.

The emerging threat has been amplified by the media coverage, which has indulged in apocalyptic worst case scenarios. This in turn has had paradoxical effects, like the hoarding and subsequent shortage of ciprofloxacin in the entire USA, followed by a rise in the stock values of its manufacturer.

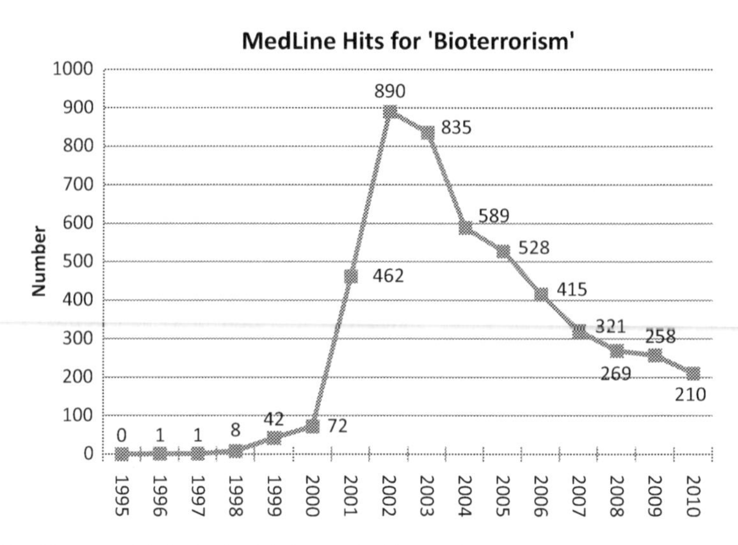

Fig. 13.2 The rise and fall of scientific interest in bioterrorism, as shown by the number of hits in the MedLine database. (Accessed 18 April 2011)

The media storm swept through the world. The anthrax scare hit the headlines and enticed the phenomenon of fake alarms: over a period of a few weeks in Italy alone there were hundreds of such alarms. Measures had to be taken immediately: A task force of experts was set up and a guideline for their management was hastily drawn. In short, the guideline instructed for a minimal and safe handling of suspicious specimens by first line operators; the heat inactivation of the material, and its referral to the national anthrax reference centre at the IZS of Foggia, where in due course the material was analyzed by PCR [8, 9, 11, 12].

Immediately after the peak of the anthrax scare, societies everywhere realized that they were unprepared to face bioterrorism. The more affluent ones allocated enormous amounts of money and implemented programmes for the early warning of biological attacks, for research on selected agents, for educating laymen and professionals, in short, for preparing for the worst. The less affluent ones, like Italy, took advantage of the growing knowledge on the threat and followed as they could.

On the judiciary side, the emergence has brought about an updating of the penal laws against the associations with the scope of terrorism in general (Law of 15 December 2001) [15], while the old penal code, Article 438, states: "Anyone who causes an epidemic through the spread of germs is punished with life imprisonment", and Article 430 states "Anyone who poisons water or substances intended for food, before they are paid or distributed for consumption, is punished with imprisonment of not less than fifteen years. If the fact is followed by death it is punished with life imprisonment". There are several other provisions for criminal offences which may occur in bioterrorism activities, and it may be recalled that in Italy all crimes must be prosecuted. Actually, this is the main difference in the response to natural epidemics and the bioterrorism threat.

13.6 Where Do We Currently Stand?

Before the anthrax scare we had to face a series of other biological emergencies, like the HIV pandemic and the Bovine Spongiform Encephalopathy. Each found Italy unprepared, and each had some strengthening effect on Italy's public health system. In particular, there was a renewed interest in infectious diseases (ID), a branch of medicine that had appeared to be superseded by antibiotics. *Ad hoc* investments led to the opening of many ID units, many more MDs embraced the specialty, and there was a flowering of mathematical models of epidemic spread. In general, these emergencies favoured the transfer into the health system of modern communication technologies.

In the last decade the SARS pandemic (2003) demonstrated the value of real time networks and of international collaboration: in a matter of weeks after the isolation of the agent by Carlo Urbani, the virus was fully characterized as a novel Coronavirus and PCR methods allowed for its detection. Italy reacted with health checks of incoming international flights, and guidelines for caring and isolating patients at two selected ID hospitals, located in the cities near Italy's two main airline hubs, where the Spallanzani Hospital (Rome) and the Sacco Hospital (Milan) are equipped with negative pressure isolation rooms, BSL-4 laboratories, and isolator ambulances and stretchers. Both are national reference centres for bio-emergency.

An urgent decree funded the establishment of a national centre for disease prevention and control, CCM, with the mission to prevent and control sanitary emergencies due to bioterrorism or incumbent epidemics [16].

In 2006 there was the first Italian report, in birds, of the highly pathogenic H5N1 influenza virus which had lingered since the 1990s in the Far East and had reached Turkey, East Europe, and Great Britain, with a number of serious human infections. The bird flu led to a stringent veterinary surveillance and to a network of dedicated laboratories. Italy followed the lead of the WHO 2005 pandemic preparedness plan, and adopted its own [25], which dictated that all Regions had to prepare similar plans, coordinating the efforts of the various agencies involved. At the central level, measures were taken as to the purchase of vaccines and antivirals, with *post factum* political controversies.

On the regulatory side, the national committee for biosafety, biotechnology and life sciences, under the patronage of the prime minister office, has drafted a code of conduct for biosafety [26] which stresses the importance of education and of strict adherence to caution in the handling of select agents.

The council of regional health assessors has agreed on a list of diseases deserving extreme surveillance and control, regardless of whether they occur naturally or maliciously. The list includes smallpox, botulism, plague, tularemia, multiple viral hemorrhagic fevers, yellow fever, Marburg virus disease, cholera, and any other quarantinable diseases considered by international authorities.

Other kinds of emergencies, like the garbage disposal crisis of Naples, the Aquila earthquake, the waves of clandestine immigrants and the recent global economic crisis have distracted from the threat of bioterrorism, which is now to be considered just one of the possible, albeit improbable, catastrophic events, for which the foundation has been laid for an integrated response. The fact that the word "bioterrorism" is not present in the national plan for health [21] nor in the national plan for prevention 2010–2012 [23] attests that it is no longer considered a priority.

13.6.1 Education for Bioterrorism

At the basis of preparedness is knowledge of the risks, first and foremost by MDs. Although some information was routinely taught about specific agents, bioterrorism was not contemplated in the university core curricula and standard textbooks, until editions published after 2002. This means that most of the physicians have had to rely on continuous medical education (CME) for training in this area. Many medical societies have included sessions on bioterrorism (and other biological emergencies) in their national congresses [34]. Some have set up study groups of experts and fostered the establishment of early warning systems and laboratory networks. The CME offer has been consistent, but its fruition has been hampered by the lack of public funding.

Universities have organized updating courses on bioterrorism and biological emergencies and have devoted postgraduate public health theses, PhD curricula, and more structured Master Courses, like the one on NBCR Medicine jointly set up by the Army and the University of Florence (see http://e-learning.med.unifi.it/didonline/anno-ii/microbiologia/MasterNBC/) which is now running its sixth edition. This Master Course is forming a highly specialized nucleus of operators, mainly military medical officers, but also public health officers in the various branches of Italy's SSN. More or less along the same line, there has been an education effort in the area of general disaster relief.

Other agencies, like the military corps of CRI (the Italian Red Cross), the DC and PC organizations, the *Corpo Nazionale dei Vigili del Fuoco* (CNVVF, the national firemen organization), or the "118" national emergency call system, have instructed their first line operators on safety issues, the correct use of equipment, and the basics of emergency interventions.

13.7 Issues About Specific Category A Agents

13.7.1 Anthrax

Natural anthrax has a long history as a public health problem in Italy, where it has been efficiently controlled by the local structures of Italy's services in the first half of the twentieth century. Extended animal vaccination, careful disposal of affected animals, and stringent veterinary surveillance have almost wiped out the disease from Italy's herds. Human cases from animal contacts have declined so much that the basic public health curricula have given less and less attention to it, relegating anthrax to be dealt with in the occupational medicine courses. Still in the 1960s a standard treatise of hygiene [27] gave a full education of anthrax and its control. Sophomore medical students exercised with *Bacillus anthracis* culture, guinea pig inoculation, and post-mortem dissection. Veterinarians on the field could perform the Ascoli reaction to diagnose anthrax in the carrions. And all provincial public health laboratories routinely tested for it, which in the Italian language had always been named *carbonchio*. In time, provincial health laboratories were dismantled, and slowly entire cohorts of MDs were formed who only had a cursory knowledge of *carbonchio*, even less of *antrace*, as the media started to call it. Hospital and territorial laboratories gradually gave up the traditional methods of diagnosis, and when the anthrax letter scares occurred, the best that could be done was to adopt a minimal guideline to safeguard first line officers.

Presently there is reasonable attention to anthrax. Regional and local health care units have done their due diligence on it and emergency and intensive care units should be ready to diagnose and treat even the pulmonary forms. A recent outbreak of natural anthrax has shown a valid integrated response to control it [14]. Small attacks would be faced similarly. False alarms are also less of a problem – one such event recently was barely reported in the local newspapers.

A massive airborne attack is considered very unlikely, but the event would considerably strain Italy's response capacity. Italy has no human vaccine, though it should have no problems with antibiotic procurement, delivery and administration. Italy would be at a loss in regard to the decontamination of large areas, and would have to rely on general plans for disasters to deal with the mass casualties.

13.7.2 Botulinum Toxin

Even natural cases of botulism are considered health emergencies, imposing immediate notification, epidemiological investigation, tracing and confiscation of incriminated foods or feeds.

In late 1996, a serious outbreak due to contamination of mascarpone cheese [2] led to centralizing the stock of anti-botulinum immune globulins and to strengthening the surveillance system.

A massive aerosol attack is considered highly improbable. Smaller attempts, like the ones in Japan by the Aum Shinrikyō sect, have been unsuccessful. Attacks to the food chain could easily overcome the treatment capacity of Italy's intensive care units, and would be faced as if they were natural outbreaks.

13.7.3 Plague

Italy has faced plague epidemics for centuries, as attested by innumerable works of art, and by historical and literary accounts. The word itself invokes terror, and *Yersinia pestis* is rightly considered in Category A, as an agent deserving priority consideration.

Again, a massive aerosol attack is considered very unlikely, but it would cause mass casualties; very many cases could be treated effectively, hospital facilities would increase to maximum capacity, but there would still be the need for domiciliary quarantine, lazarettos, travel restrictions and the like. Limited attacks, say a number of contagious cases going through airline hubs, should be spotted by international warning networks and ensuing outbreaks be confined and controlled.

13.7.4 Smallpox

Universal vaccination had been compulsory in Italy. Suspended in 1977, it was definitely abrogated in 1981, but pediatricians had already discontinued it a number of years before. Perhaps those over 50 years (about half of the total population) [30] have in fact been vaccinated and might have some residual immunity to smallpox.

In 2002, following the third ministerial meeting on health security and bioterrorism, the Minister of Health announced that Italy has a national stockpile of five million doses of the traditional vaccine, that could be diluted to vaccinate twenty-five million persons. He also stated that Italy has no hyper-immune gamma globulins and announced the intention to buy a stock of the antiviral cidofovir [6] for the treatment of about 500 cases [22]. In addition, there was a pledge for an education effort, such that "every emergency room doctor or nurse will be prepared to recognize a smallpox case".

Clearly we have to rely on the international intelligence cooperation in order to assess the risk of a return of smallpox. The remote idea that it could appear in Italy is appalling, in the light of what happened following its introduction in countries which had been free from it for decades [33], as in Yugoslavia in 1972. In the event that smallpox be reintroduced, the DC and PC structures would be alerted and emergency legislation would be passed to limit civil rights and enforce containment of the epidemic.

13.7.5 Tularemia

Tularemia is not enzoonotic in Italy, but it has been repeatedly introduced with wild game, giving rise to small human outbreaks. Of interest is the one in Tuscany, where cases were due to contamination of small spring water reservoirs.

A serious aerosol attack would be undetected until cases were taken for emergency care and would be correctly diagnosed by hospital laboratories, of which the smaller ones would not attempt culture methods, because of the lack of BSL-3 facilities. Pneumonias would be treated with an empirical antibiotic therapy, and standard isolation could be guaranteed.

13.7.6 Hemorrhagic Viral Fevers

Attention to exotic hemorrhagic viral fevers (HVF) is driven by the fear that they could be imported by the normal travel routes and mass illegal immigration rather than by the threat of bioterrorism. Two hospitals have been earmarked as appropriate to manage them, and are equipped to strictly isolate the patients and to diagnose HVF in BSL-4 laboratories.

13.7.7 Category B Agents

Italy's physicians and veterinarians are knowledgeable about Q fever and brucellosis. Hospitals and laboratories are well equipped for their diagnosis and treatment, and ASLs could perform adequate epidemiological enquiries.

Not so for glanders and melioidosis, the first having long disappeared from the medical core curricula, the second having never been seen in Italy. In the unlikely event of their malicious use, diagnosis of human cases would be delayed, and therapy would be empirical.

Of the biological toxins in Category B, the staphylococcal enterotoxin B is well known for occasional food poisoning outbreaks, which are managed routinely; somewhat less adequately when *C. perfringens* toxin is involved. An attack by aerosol is considered less feasible. In the event, Italy would be unprepared to detect it immediately.

Ricin toxin is more of a problem. The raw material is easily acquired, the toxin may be prepared by an individual or by a small organization, and attempts to prepare it have been discovered in several countries. Dispersal of the powder form, either by mailings or otherwise, would go undetected in the absence of warnings. Cases would be taken to emergency rooms, many of which are linked to poison centres.

13.7.8 Category C Agents

Viruses in this category are not present in Italy, as they are exotic and/or emergent. Cases would be managed by ID specialists, with limited laboratory help for specific diagnosis and no specific therapies. Vaccination for yellow fever is normally offered to travellers, and should be available if needed.

As to the extremely drug-resistant *Mycobacterium tuberculosis* (XDR-TB), there had been a long period of complacency, during which the traditional complex structure for tuberculosis control was dismantled in Italy, although there has been the realization that it is still a problem, as it is reintroduced by immigrants from endemic areas, and standard treatments are often ineffective. Interest in *Mycobacteria* has recently increased, and Italy has a network of reference laboratories which have implemented modern techniques for identification and drug sensitivity assays. Attention to XDR-TB [29] is high on account of its natural history.

13.7.9 Other Agents

The official lists are not exhaustive of the agents that may be exploited for bioterrorism. Indeed, it would be easier for a malicious layman to get hold of *Amanita phalloides* and to serve it at a banquet than, say, to organize an attack with a *Brucella* or a *Coxiella* organism.

Regarding food and feed safety, the threat can only be faced by a general awareness of the risk. In Italy, the plan for crisis management in the field is the State-Regions Agreement of 24 January 2008, drawn in actuation of European directives, which provides for the establishment, in case of an emergency, of national, regional, and local crisis units. Like several similar regulations, this has a clause stating that no new funds are provided.

13.8 Closing Remarks

The threat of bioterrorism still lingers as a menace to public health and to society in general. Its emergence has had wide-ranging effects on the internal organization of advanced countries, which are now more prepared to face it, and can rely on international collaboration and mutual aid. In Italy, the mainstay for the response to a biological attack is represented by the public health system, entrusted to Italy's national health service. As elsewhere, other more recent biological emergencies have had priority consideration, strengthening the response capacity of public health, and of society in general, particularly in the areas of education, training, and integrated planning.

References

1. Alfani G, Melegaro A (2010), Pandemie d'Italia. Dalla peste nera all'influenza suina: l'impatto sulla società. Egea. ISBN/EAN: 9788823832664
2. Aureli P, Di Cunto M, Maffei A, De Chiara G, Franciosa G, Accorinti L, Gambardella AM, Greco D (2000) An outbreak in Italy of botulism associated with a dessert made with mascarpone cream cheese. Eur J Epidemiol 16(10):913–918
3. B.W. Reports (Intel) (1996) Italian experiments in BW, by named scientists: the national archives: WO 188/685 C411857
4. Berlinguer G (2011) Storia della salute. Da privilegio a diritto. Giunti Editore. ISBN-13: 9788809053656
5. Cosmacini G (2005) Storia della medicina e della sanità in Italia. Dalla peste nera ai giorni nostri. Laterza. ISBN-13:9788842077671

6. De Clercq E (2002) Cidofovir in the treatment of poxvirus infections, Antiviral Research, 55(1): 1–13. http://www.sciencedirect.com/science?_ob=MImg&_imagekey=B6T2H-45578G7-1-W&_cdi=4919&_user=8746464&_pii=S0166354202000086&_origin=brow se&_coverDate=07%2F31%2F2002&_sk=999449998&view=c&wchp=dGLbVtz-zSkW A&md5=5be36e880b35de5b894524948bbb814c&ie=/sdarticle.pdf. Accessed 22 Mar 2011
7. Di Feo G (2009) Veleni di Stato. BUR Rizzoli
8. Drago L, de Vecchi E, Lombardi A, Nicola L, Valli M, Gismondo MR (2002) Bactericidal activity of levofloxacin, gatifloxacin, penicillin, meropenem and rokitamycin against Bacillus anthracis clinical isolates. JAC 50(6):1059–1063
9. Drago L, Lombardi A, de Vecchi E, Gismondo MR (2002) Real-time PCR assay for rapid detection of Bacillus anthracis spores in clinical samples. J Clin Microbiol 40(11):4399
10. European Commission (2010) Humanitarian Aid & Civil Protection. Italy – Emergency planning. http://ec.europa.eu/echo/civil_protection/civil/vademecum/it/2-it-2.html. Accessed 20 Mar 2011
11. Fasanella A (2003) The test to reveal anthrax spores in suspect specimens in Italy. Lesson of 2001 Anthrax episode – Oral special session. In: Proceedings of the 5th international conference on anthrax, Nice (France)
12. Fasanella A, Losito S, Adone R, Ciuchini F, Trotta T, Altamura SA, Chiocco D, Ippolito G (2003) PCR assay to detect Bacillus anthracis spores in heat-treated specimens. J Clin Microbiol 41:896–899
13. Giannattasio P (2002) Libro Bianco 2002. Ministero della Difesa. http://files.studiperlapace.it/spp_zfiles/docs/20060816165432.pdf. Accessed 15 Mar 2011
14. Kreidl P, Stifter E, Richter A, Aschbachert R, Nienstedt F, Unterhuber H, Barone S, Huemer HP, Carattoli A, Moroder L, Ciofi Degli Atti ML, Rota MC, Morosetti G, Larcher C (2006) Anthrax in animals and a farmer in Alto Adige, Italy. Euro Surveill 11(7):pii=2900. http://www.eurosurveillance.org/ViewArticle.aspx?ArticleId=2900
15. Law 15 December 2001, n. 438, Conversione in legge, con modificazioni, del decreto-legge 18 ottobre 2001, n. 374, recante disposizioni urgenti per contrastare il terrorismo internazionale". Gazzetta Ufficiale N. 293 del 18 dicembre 2001. http://www.camera.it/parlam/leggi/01438l.htm. Accessed 15 Apr 2011
16. Law 26 May 2004, n.138: Conversione in legge, con modificazioni, del decreto-legge 29 marzo 2004, n. 81, recante interventi urgenti per fronteggiare situazioni di pericolo per la salute pubblica. Gazzetta Ufficiale N. 125 del 29 Maggio 2004. http://www.ccm-network.it/documenti_Ccm/normativa/L_138-2004.pdf
17. Law 24 February 1992, n. 225: Istituzione del Servizio nazionale della protezione civile. http://www.protezionecivile.it/cms/attach/editor/225_1992.pdf. Accessed 20 Apr 2011
18. Lo Scalzo A, Donatini A, Orzella L, Cicchetti A, Profili S, Maresso A (2009) Italy: health system review. Health Syst Transit 11(6):1–216
19. Marmo F, Urbano F (2008) L'innovazione Tecnologica del Servizio Sanitario dell'Esercito nelle Attività Campali. Presentation at the meeting 'Soccorso integrato nelle maxi emergenze', Florence, 15–17 May 2008
20. Mennonna G (1958) Limiti della partecipazione della sanità militare al programma di difesa civile nel nostro paese. Minerva med 49(63–64):3067–3069
21. Ministero della Salute (2005) Piano Sanitario Nazionale 2006–2008. http://www.salute.gov.it/resources/static/primopiano/316/PSN_2006_08_28_marzo.pdf. Accessed 24 Mar 2011
22. Ministero della Salute (2006) Rapporto sulle cose fatte 2001–2005. http://issuu.com/dariogalvagno/docs/ministerosalute_rapportosullecosefatte. Accessed 26 Mar 2011
23. Ministero della Salute (2010) Piano nazionale della prevenzione 2010–2012. http://www.salute.gov.it/imgs/C_17_pubblicazioni_1384_allegato.pdf. Accessed 1 Mar 2011
24. Ministero della Salute (2011) Annuario Statistico del Servizio Sanitario Nazionale, Anno 2008. http://www.salute.gov.it/imgs/C_17_pubblicazioni_1488_allegato.pdf. Accessed 14 Apr 2011
25. Piano Nazionale di Preparazione e Risposta ad una Pandemia Influenzale (2005). http://www.salute.gov.it/imgs/C_17_pubblicazioni_501_allegato.pdf
26. Presidenza del Consiglio dei Ministri, Comitato Nazionale per la Biosicurezza, le Biotecnologie e le Scienze della Vita (2010) Codice di Condotta per la Biosicurezza. http://www.governo.it/biotecnologie/documenti/Codici_condotta_biosicurezza.pdf

27. Puntoni V (1962–1964) Trattato d'Igiene, Tumminelli Editore
28. Snowden FM (2006) Nazism and bioterror in the Pontine marshes. In: The conquest of malaria: Italy, 1900–1962. Yale University Press, New Haven. ISBN 13: 978–0300108996
29. Sotgiu G, Centis R, D'ambrosio L, De Lorenzo S, D'arcy Richardson M, Lange C, Manissero D, Migliori GB (2010) TBNET MDR-TB project: development of a standardised tool to survey MDR-/XDR-TB case management in Europe. Eur Respir J 36(1):208–211
30. Statistiche demografiche ISTAT: Official data on residing population (2010). http://demo.istat.it/pop2010/index.html
31. Stephenson J (1996) Confronting a biological Armageddon: experts tackle prospect of bioterrorism. JAMA 276(5):349–351
32. Urbano F (2006) Alle basi del Bioterrorismo: un approccio storico alla Guerra Biologica. Caleidoscopio, 38, 3–138. ISSN 1120–6756. http://www.formazioneesicurezza.it/AA_SPECIALISTICA/Dispense/A2%20-%20Scienze%20della%20prevenzione%20applicate/02%20-%20Malattie%20infettive/A2%20-%20Urbano%20-%20Bioterrorismo.pdf. Accessed 1 Mar 2011
33. Urbano F (2011) Gli ultimi colpi di coda del vaiolo. http://e-learning.med.unifi.it/didonline/anno-ii/microbiologia/MasterNBC/PPT/GliUltimiColpiDiCodaDelVaiolo.PPT. Accessed 14 Apr 2011
34. Urbano P, Urbano F (2004) Le nuove emergenze: il bioterrorismo. Microbiol Med 19:120–121 ISSN: 1120–0146
35. Wadman M (1997) Action needed to counter bioterrorism. Nature 388(6644):703
36. World Health Organization (2010) World health statistics. ISBN 978 92 4 156398. http://www.who.int/whosis/whostat/EN_WHS10_TOCintro.pdf. Accessed 1 Apr 2011

Chapter 14
Case Study – Poland

Anna Bielecka and Janusz Kocik

Abstract A high rate of morbidity and/or death, fear and panic, and economic losses are just some of the consequences of both, natural and deliberate releases of highly contagious diseases. Epidemiological surveillance, rapid outbreak detection, infectious agent identification, response and recovery, including decontamination activities, are able to minimize the risk of a biological incident. Inter-departmental cooperation – public administration authorities, civil and military services – might also reduce the effects of biological threats. This chapter presents the crisis management system used by the Polish government in the case of a natural epidemic of a dangerous infectious disease or a bioterrorist attack. The supportive role and capabilities of military institutions are also discussed.

14.1 Introduction

In Poland, according to the National Institute of Public Health reports, the most common illnesses are gastrointestinal infections of viral and bacterial etiology, with the incidence per 100,000 population in 2009 of 86.0 and 28.4 respectively. Influenza and influenza-like illness are frequent as well, but less than 0.9% of all cases required hospitalization in 2009.

Regarding human infectious diseases and zoonoses likely to be used as biological weapon agents, only single cases of anthrax, botulism, tularemia, Q fever, dengue fever, leptospirosis, and brucellosis have been reported. Most of these were imported to Poland from endemic regions. Cholera, plague, glanders, diphtheria, smallpox, SARS, as well as West Nile fever, yellow fever, and viral hemorrhagic fever cases have not been reported [1].

A. Bielecka (✉) • J. Kocik
Department of Epidemiology, Military Institute of Hygiene and Epidemiology, Warsaw, Poland
e-mail: abielecka@wihe.waw.pl; jkocik@wihe.waw.pl

I. Hunger et al. (eds.), *Biopreparedness and Public Health: Exploring Synergies*, NATO Science for Peace and Security Series A: Chemistry and Biology,
DOI 10.1007/978-94-007-5273-3_14,

Recent trends in terrorist attacks indicate that apart from conventional weapons, we face the threat of unconventional hostilities, such as those using weapons of mass destruction (WMD).

The progressive development of the biosciences provides immense positive social, economic and health benefits to our society. Nevertheless, their development provides dangerous opportunities for potential perpetrators (the "dual-use" research aspect), as well.

An intentional biological attack (bioterrorist act) and a coincidental infectious diseases case (epidemic) evoke similar emergency situations. Efficient management by public administration in association with civil and military institutions is the key aspect of good governance. Furthermore, their mutual cooperation may improve the first response to the threat and reduce its detrimental effects on people and the environment.

14.2 Biosafety and Biosecurity in Poland

In accordance with Article 4 of the Biological and Toxin Weapons Convention (BTWC), each Member State is obliged to take the necessary steps to prohibit and prevent the spread of biological agents, toxins, weapons, equipment and means of delivery within the State or in any place under its jurisdiction. Poland is committed to this obligation, but activities towards its fulfillment are indirect and encompassed by actions taken for different reasons, like public health safety.

In April 2005, the Minister of Health promulgated the regulation regarding rules for working with dangerous pathogens and health protection for the professionals exposed to these agents (biosafety measures, classification of the facilities). This piece of legislation is a direct implementation of European Parliament Directive 2000/54/WE. In 2002, based on the Act on Genetically Modified Organisms enacted in 2001, the Minister of Environmental Protection issued the regulation comprising lists of agents grouped in risk categories and the corresponding containment levels of biosafety measures in laboratories in which work with these agents is being conducted. These two pieces of legislation provide the framework for security of agents of concern through establishment of access controls required from the safety point of view.

Polish legislation still lacks specific legal measures in order to reduce the probability of a biological attack through improved security of microbial collections and laboratories. A national laboratory register and personnel and pathogen accountability have not been undertaken in a coordinated manner. There is a general understanding that biosafety measures are sufficient to prevent misuse of the agents although there are opinions that some additional measures concerning the handling of pathogens should be considered.

Currently, Poland is actively engaged in the creation of new instruments for the fight against terrorism and ensuring global biosafety and biosecurity. The national BTWC Implementation Working Group, consisting of policy makers and representatives of the scientific community and law authorities, has prepared a draft legal Act, in which legislative and regulatory issues under the BTWC will be enclosed. The Act will be in force in the end of 2012.

14.3 Biopreparedness and Response Measures in Poland

The term "biopreparedness" is used for the complex of anticipated measures regarding bioterrorism taken from the EC's Green Paper on Bio-Preparedness [2] in which it is stated that the term "preparedness" is used in a generic way and covers all aspects such as prevention, protection, first response capacity, prosecution of criminals/terrorists, surveillance, research capacity, response, and recovery. The term also covers the steps taken to diminish the threat of deliberate contamination of the food supply with biological agents and to protect against biological warfare [3, 4].

The administrative and operational framework for the protection of the population in Poland in the case of a biological incident is secured by the following acts: (1) The Constitution of the Republic of Poland of 2 April 1997 stipulates that in situations of particular danger, if ordinary constitutional measures are inadequate, any of the following appropriate extraordinary measures may be introduced: martial law, a state of emergency, or a state of natural disaster, (2) The Crisis Management Act of 26 April 2007 specifies the authorities responsible for crisis management, their tasks and the general principles for crisis management, and (3) The Act on the State of Natural Disaster of 18 April 2002 specifies the conditions for implementing extraordinary measures in case of disasters, which may be either natural or deliberate. The Act provides definitions, rights of and restrictions on the public during a state of disaster, specifies the authorities responsible for implementing tasks, and sets out general principles for consequence management.

Poland has implemented an inter-sectorial system that would be engaged in the management of the consequences of biological weapons use, through strengthening communication systems and division of tasks among the public administration institutions (see Fig. 14.1).

The Cabinet headed by the Prime Minister ensures internal security and public order in Poland. The Cabinet urges recommendations and updates or changes in regulations regarding planning and implementation of defence preparation tasks, and identifies objects important for national security and defence.

The Governmental Security Center is directly responsible for the governmental coordination of inter-sectorial response and crisis management at the national level. The institution was established in 2008 and is subordinated directly to the Prime Minister. The Ministry of Interior, the Ministry of Health with its subordinate institution, the Chief Sanitary Inspectorate, the Polish National Police, the National Headquarters of the State Fire Service, the National Border Guard Headquarters, the State Sanitary Inspectorate, the Military Sanitary Inspection of the Ministry of National Defence, and scientific institutes such as the Military Institute of Hygiene and Epidemiology and the National Institute for Public Health – National Institute

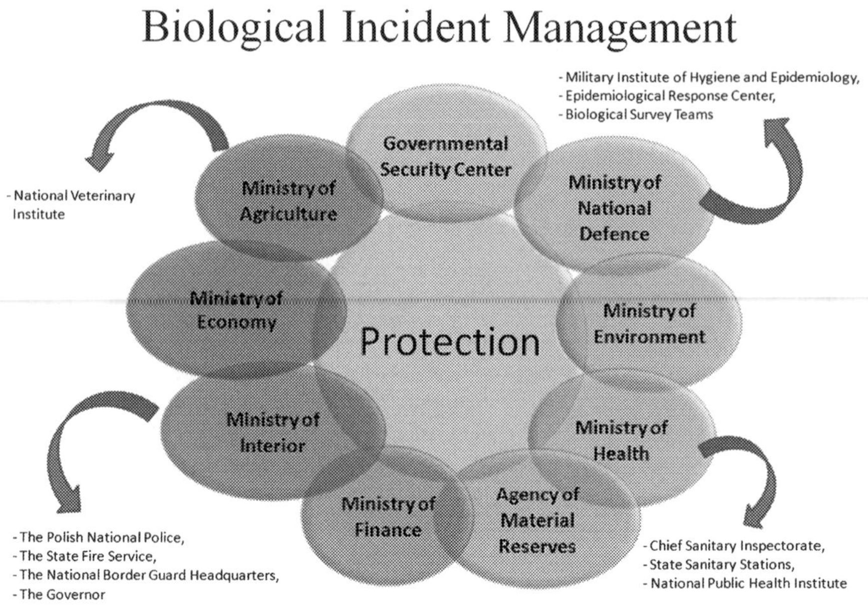

Fig. 14.1 Biological incident management system in Poland

of Hygiene are major players that undertake coordination actions in the case of a biological attack or unusual outbreak. The network for communication and operating procedures for foreseeable scenarios such as "white powder" hoaxes had been established after the 2001 anthrax attacks in the USA.

14.3.1 The Supportive Role of the Polish Armed Forces

The supreme authority of state administration competent for the defence of the State is the Minister of National Defence, who supervises defence tasks realized by the government, state bodies and institutions. In addition, under the Act of 30 May 1996, the Minister is also obliged to ensure defence and national security via mobilization of reserve materials.

In case of an infectious disease threat and/or a bioterrorism attack the Minister of National Defence mobilizes the appropriate military units specialized in health care management and coordination.

The Polish Armed Forces play a supportive role in response to biological events due to both, highly contagious disease outbreaks and bioterrorism acts. The military has its own system to ensure anti-epidemic protection of soldiers, namely an epidemic surveillance and reporting system including detection capabilities, clinical and/or environmental sample collection, preliminary/rapid diagnostic testing for agent identification, measures to secure an area and the infective material, transport procedures, and final confirmation capability conducted in the BSL-3 reference laboratory at the Military Institute of Hygiene and Epidemiology (MIHE). In case of a biological incident, the Minister of National Defence instantaneously mobilizes competent individuals able to eliminate the harmful effects and perform surrounding decontamination.

The Military Health Care Inspectorate is the primary institution responsible for military health care for both troops deployed in the country and those in abroad mission service. The Polish Armed Forces Military Sanitary Inspection supports the Inspectorate in relation to outbreak surveillance. The Military Sanitary Inspection conducts sanitary situation monitoring, preventive medicine and disease control, epidemiological surveillance, medical investigation, and countermeasures against the use of CBRN (chemical, biological, radiological, nuclear) agents.

14.3.2 Surveillance

Disease surveillance is carried out by the national epidemiological system. The State Sanitary Inspection System collects data on a number of reportable diseases (as set down by the Infectious Diseases Act of 2008 and the International Health Regulations, WHO) from health care and state sanitary inspection laboratories. The information is centrally analyzed in the National Public Health Institute.

The diseases reportable under the Infectious Diseases Act are retrospectively analyzed by the National Public Health Institute. Outbreaks are investigated by the State Sanitary Inspection. Active surveillance is feasible through this system, including case and contact tracing, once a case definition is established and the disease is determined to pose an imminent threat to life (like meningococcal encephalitis). No syndrome-based system of surveillance is used. The system is not real-time, but has a descriptive and lessons-learned value.

The Chief Sanitary Inspectorate, with its Anti-Epidemic Department and subordinate system of the State Sanitary Inspection, is responsible for the institution of control measures (e.g. restriction on public gatherings, sanitary cordon, etc.).

Measures regulating crisis communication (nation level, and with EU) are initiated by the Health Security Committee under ECDC recommendations, promulgated by focal points located in key national institutions. The International Health Regulations Point of Contact (IHR POC) is placed in the National Public Health Institute. The Early Warning and Response System Point of Contact (EWRS POC) and the European Centre for Disease Prevention and Control Point of Contact (ECDC POC) are situated in the Chief Sanitary Inspectorate. The points of contact for the Rapid Alert System – Biological and Chemical Attacks and Threats (RAS-BICHAT POC) and the European Union Health Security Committee (EC HSC POC) are established in the Department of Defence Affairs of the Ministry of Health. The World Health Organization Point of Contact (WHO POC) is also placed in the Ministry of Health.

As mentioned above, the Armed Forces have their own system. The data are collected from military treatment facilities and through the Military Preventive Medicine Centers. The Army used to report to the NATO Epidemiological Reporting System as long as it existed. Now the Polish Armed Forces are looking forward to the establishment of the NATO Deployment Health Surveillance Centre, part of the NATO MilMed Centre of Excellence.

14.3.3 Measures Related to Food and Feed Protection, Animal Health Protection, Plant Protection, and the Environment

Routine measures are undertaken by the State Veterinary and Phytosanitary Inspection concerning food security, animal health and plant protection. Hazard Analysis and Critical Control Point (HACCP) measures are observed. No specific measures are undertaken against the possible use of animal and plant pathogens as a means of warfare. Adequate measures for diagnostics for animal and plant diseases and control measures against the spread of disease (e.g. culling animals) have been practiced in natural outbreaks and the response system and public information policy have proven to be effective in public affairs caused by influenza H5N1 and foot and mouth disease outbreaks. The regulation issued by the Minister of Health in 2006 established close cooperation among the State Sanitary Inspection, the Veterinary Inspection, and the Ministry of Environmental Protection in the management of outbreaks of several zoonotic diseases including anthrax, tularemia, and Q fever which are considered potential biological weapon agents.

14.3.4 The First Response

The general practitioner (GP) first recognizes symptoms among patients. Once a GP diagnoses a potentially dangerous disease or an infectious disease which arouses his/her suspicion he/she is obligated to report the event to the County Sanitary Inspector. The County Sanitary Inspector informs the local Crisis Management Center, the local Police, the local Fire Service, an appropriate local director of a hospital, and the Provincial Sanitary Inspection. Further steps in the notification of an unnatural event are like a reaction chain, in which the local service representatives report to authorities on the regional level, and finally to the central level according to the scheme set out in Fig. 14.2.

The National Consultant on Communicable Disease Control has issued guidelines for hospitals concerning the management of a patient suspected of being infected with a dangerous disease. The guidelines also relate to people having been in direct contact with a potentially infected person. Dealing with dead bodies is governed by national health provisions.

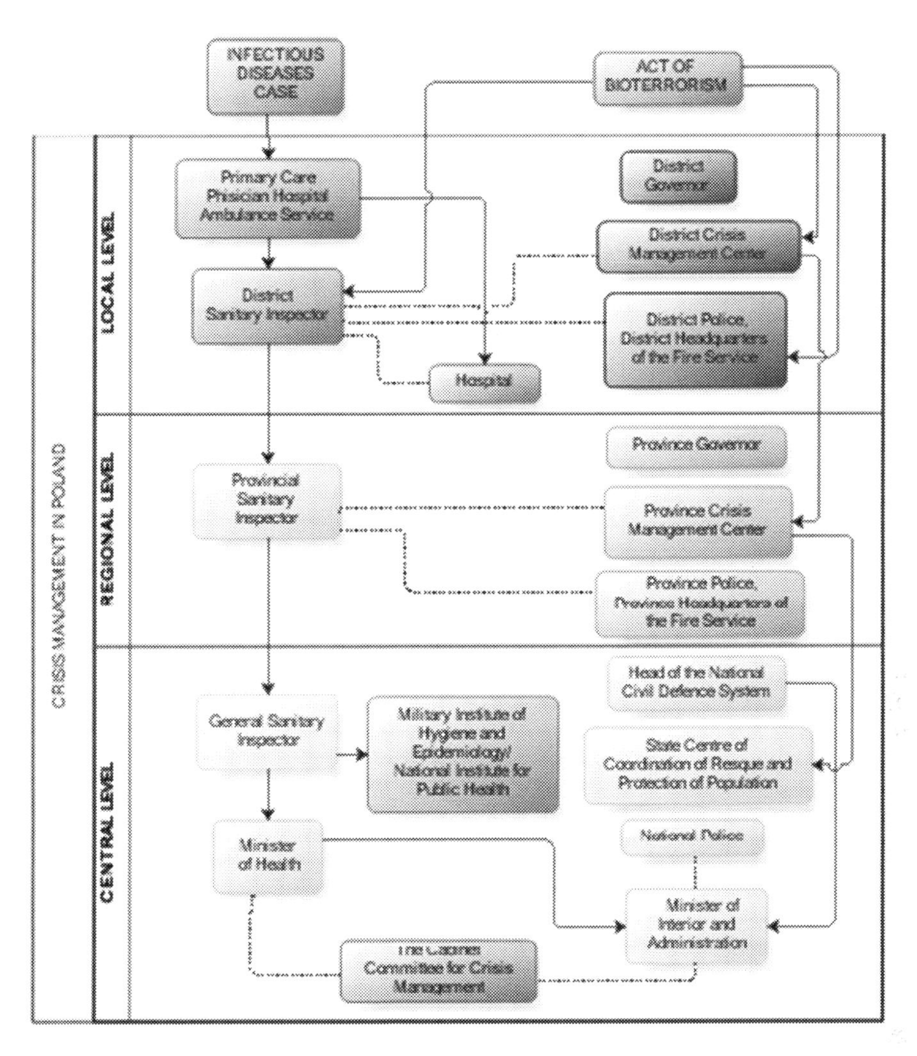

Fig. 14.2 Notification and information sharing at the local, regional and national level

14.3.5 Detection and Identification Capabilities

The capability to detect and identify biological agents in the field after a bio-attack was originally developed by specialists from MIHE. In 2001, the Head of the Military Health Care Inspectorate created seven Biological Survey Teams, including two in research centres in MIHE, and from January 2003, in military preventive medicine centres in Bydgoszcz, Gdynia, Krakow, Wroclaw, and Modlin. Later, the dedicated military unit – the Epidemiological Response Centre – was established by the Polish Armed Forces with the primary responsibility to react to

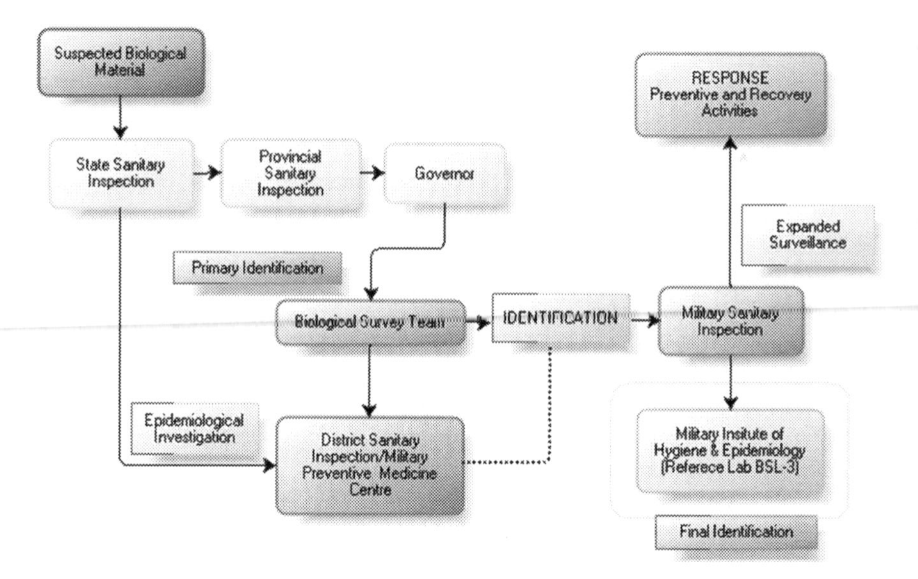

Fig. 14.3 In situ detection and identification of biological agents

biological outbreaks with mobile detection capabilities, sampling in high containment individual protection equipment, and decontamination. All teams are capable of primary detection of biological agents in environmental samples (Fig. 14.3).

14.3.6 The Research Capacity

The confirmed identification of selected biological agents that are on the list of most probable biological weapon agents is possible at the BSL-3 microbiological laboratory at MIHE's Biological Threats Identification and Countermeasure Centre in Pulawy. MIHE's mission is to conduct scientific research, diagnosis, prophylaxis, surveillance, training and services associated with medical protection and countermeasures against the use of weapons of mass destruction (WMD). It is a unique research centre for this purpose in Poland. Apart from that, the Institute is providing expertise in the fields of hygiene, epidemiology, microbiology, pharmacology, toxicology, radiobiology and radiation protection, applied and nutritional physiology, and veterinary sciences. The biodefence research, the biological weapon agent diagnostics, and the medical countermeasures development is carried out with support of the European Defence Agency, the US Defense Advanced Research Projects Agency, the Polish Ministry of Defence and the Polish Ministry of Science and Higher Education.

MIHE is the key institution active in biosecurity in Poland. It helps the administration to develop dual-use research monitoring activities and the national crisis management procedures for outbreaks of highly contagious diseases, whether natural or deliberate. MIHE follows activities at the BTWC, WHO, EU, UN and other international institutions directed against biological weapons and the bioterrorism threat, as well as developments of medical aspects of CBRN defence in NATO. Currently, MIHE participates in the implementation of the education programme for PhD students in the life sciences, which includes aspects of microbiology, epidemiology, bioethics, bioterrorism, and strategic planning.

Other institutions like the National Public Health Institute and civilian State Sanitary Stations in several major cities are capable of diagnostics at the confirmatory level in terms of biosafety standards, but these types of diagnostics are not part of their daily routine.

Veterinary samples may be tested under high containment in the National Veterinary Institute in Pulawy.

14.3.7 Consequence Management Capabilities

Measures to reduce the vulnerability of the population to an attack through ensuring adequate supplies of vaccines as well as stores of protective equipment have been undertaken. The stockpile of respiratory masks and individual protection equipment is sufficient for initial operations and can be mobilized as needed. Mobile decontamination equipment is stockpiled in a national reserve, but fire servicemen have responsibility for this type of equipment as well. The strategic stockpile of pharmaceuticals and vaccines is managed by the Agency of Material Reserve.

The Department for Defence Affairs in the Ministry of Health is responsible for planning, coordination, and organization of resources and capabilities for hospital preparedness for mass casualties or in-house surge capacity and quarantine/isolation capacity.

Typically, once consecutive public health threats emerge, the general rule is to plan medical countermeasure availability in quantities to at least secure first responders, medical personnel and risk groups in the general population.

Specifically designed medical centres were adapted for patient reception in the case of a bioterrorism attack. With this goal in mind, the containment level in several infectious disease clinics and hospitals were upgraded and the primary institution of this type is the State Infectious Disease Hospital in the capital city of Warsaw. New emergency rooms are frequently furnished with limited decontamination capabilities.

14.3.8 Training of the Responsible Personnel

The organization of response has been trained and practiced in mock exercises at both the internal and European levels. Coordination has also been thoroughly exercised in reality during pandemic influenza activities through the coordinated actions of the Polish Pandemic Committee that were undertaken within the Polish National Pandemic Plan. Military mobile sampling, detection and identification capabilities have been exercised in humanitarian support missions concentrated around the investigation of influenza like illness cases in Lviv Oblast in Western Ukraine in 2009.

Training activities, considered part of many international initiatives focused on biosafety and biosecurity, are also provided. Currently, MIHE supports the enhancement of biosafety in the Ukrainian Anti-Plague Station in Simferopol (Autonomous Republic of Crimea) sponsored by the European Commission's Threat Reduction Programme.

14.3.9 Response

Emergency institutions, such as the Fire Service, the Police, the Emergency Health Service, and the Public Health Service have been trained, to some extent, in managing communications, securing scenes, decontamination, and administering first aid during hoaxes and credible events. Individual case management and public health control measures are being addressed in education programmes in medical universities. The State Sanitary Inspection held a series of intensive train-the-trainer courses. Currently, the knowledge is transferred to the trainees through e-learning activities.

In case of a catastrophic incident, most of the regional hospitals are capable to provide primary medical care. The containment levels in several infectious disease clinics and hospitals were upgraded, one of the leading being the State Infectious Disease Hospital in the capital city of Warsaw. New emergency rooms are frequently furnished with limited decontamination capabilities.

Communication and liaison plans for bioterrorism events were expanded. Specific plans and templates for highly communicable disease outbreaks – e.g. a case study on smallpox – were developed for use by the administration at the state and local levels and included quarantine, isolation and decontamination procedures.

Practical exercises – New Watchman, Common Ground, and Aeolus – have been recently conducted. The major lessons identified were improving communication, delineating the scope of responsibilities of different administration institutions where fields superimpose, and improving the level of coordination.

14.3.10 Recovery

The main aim of the recovery phase is to restore the afflicted area to its previous state. Recovery efforts are about issues and decisions that must be made after identifying needs. Recovery efforts are concerned with rebuilding destroyed property, re-employment, and the repair of essential infrastructure.

Measures for joint investigations, evidence collection, and logistics have not been spelled out. A clear communication and media management policy in order to forestall and prevent mass panic has not been prepared specifically for a bioterrorism attack. Nevertheless, previously conducted exercises have shown that general media management rules may be sufficiently effective.

14.4 Concluding Remarks

Emergency management committees and working groups may differ by name and organization from country to country, but there is a common groundwork of concepts and principles upon which they ought to operate. Emergency management strategies and activities need to be flexible and adaptable within the overall comprehensive and integrated approaches not only due to diverse range of hazards and communities, but also due to environmental factors. The approach to emergency management policy and decision making needs to be coherent. It is well known that working together with communities, governments, and all key stakeholders is essential to achieve a cooperative and supportive approach to implementing emergency management programmes.

References

1. Czarkowski M, Cielebąk E, Kondej B, Staszewska E (2010) Infectious diseases and poisonings in Poland in 2009. Warsaw: National Institute of Public Health, Chief Sanitary Inspectorate. www.pzh.gov.pl/oldpage/epimeld/2009/Ch_2009.pdf
2. European Commission (2007) Green paper on bio-preparedness, COM(2007) 399 final. http://ec.europa.eu/food/resources/gp_bio_preparedness_en.pdf
3. European Union (2009) Council Regulation (EC) No 428/2009 of 5 May 2009, Off J Eur Union L 134/1. http://trade.ec.europa.eu/doclib/docs/2009/June/tradoc_143390.pdf
4. Ministry of Economy (2000) Polish legal basis for control of foreign goods, technologies and services of strategic importance. http://www.mg.gov.pl/Gospodarka/DKE/Akty/obrotzagranica#

Chapter 15
Case Study – Romania

Alexandru Rafila and Daniela Pitigoi

Abstract Countering bioterrorism, as other health threats caused by infectious agents, requires good preparedness, and early warning and response, which can be achieved by an efficient epidemiological surveillance system. In 1990, Romania inherited a functional and quite efficient epidemiological surveillance system from the former communist regime, based on pyramidal and autocratic principles where the state control was absolute. In 2001, the assessment conducted by WHO/Europe showed many unsatisfactory elements of the remaining epidemiological surveillance system for communicable diseases, with a lack of procedures, poor microbiology laboratory capacities, and overlapping responsibilities. The lack of a coordinating body was evident, especially during bioterrorist threats following 9/11 attacks in New York. In 2003 and 2004, the PHARE Project offered an important opportunity for Romania to improve the Romanian System of Epidemiological Surveillance and Control of Communicable Diseases. At the end of this project many of the technical capacities had been improved, specialized trainings of epidemiologists and microbiologists were carried out, and a coordinating body of the epidemiological surveillance network was established [1]. Furthermore, a National Plan of Action was approved by the Minister of Health with the declared objective to improve the system in order to comply with EU standards. At present, the National Institute of Public Health hosts the National Center for Communicable Diseases Surveillance and Control which coordinates the epidemiological network and serves as the

A. Rafila (✉)
Clinic II, Microbiology,University of Medicine and Pharmacy "Carol Davila", Bucharest, Romania

National Institute for Infectious Diseases "Prof. Dr. Matei Bals", Bucharest, Romania
e-mail: arafila@yahoo.com

D. Pitigoi
National Institute for Infectious Diseases "Prof. Dr. Matei Bals", Clinic II, Microbiology, Bucharest, Romania

I. Hunger et al. (eds.), *Biopreparedness and Public Health: Exploring Synergies*,
NATO Science for Peace and Security Series A: Chemistry and Biology,
DOI 10.1007/978-94-007-5273-3_15,

Romanian focal point for international institutions such as WHO and ECDC. Each year, comprehensive reports regarding surveillance in Romania of many communicable diseases are published, including diseases potentially related to bioterrorism. Until now, no evidence of a bioterrorism event has been registered in Romania.

15.1 Introduction

Regarding the global impact of public health emergencies at the international level, communicable diseases are a top priority and countries need to develop a modern system of surveillance and control of outbreaks. This has also been a priority of the public health authorities in Romania in the last 10 years and important steps have been taken in order to develop an epidemiological surveillance system based on EU standards, integrated in a national emergency system [2].

15.2 Overview

Romania is a medium sized EU member state, with the ninth largest territory, and the seventh largest population. The country has an area of 238,391 km^2 and an estimated population of 21.5 million people (2009) with a density of 90 people per km^2.

From the administrative point of view the country is divided in 41 counties and the capital Bucharest. Each county has its own administrative structures including those for health and emergencies.

Demographic indicators from 2008 showed a negative growth of population and a relatively high infant mortality, compared to other EU member states. The birth rate is 10.3 per 1,000 inhabitants, the general mortality is 11.8 per 1,000 inhabitants. The infant mortality is 11 per 1,000 live births, but with a decreasing trend. Life expectancy is 73.3 years (69.7 years for men and 77.4 years for women). The main diseases as causes of death are listed in Table 15.1.

Table 15.1 Main diseases as causes of death in Romania in 2008 (per 100,000 inhabitants)

Main diseases as causes of death	Men	Women
Cardiovascular disease	696.2	727.2
Cancer	264.4	170.3
Gastrointestinal	89.0	55.6
Respiratory	75.4	40.0
Infectious	17.5	5.9
Tuberculosis	12.8	2.7

Table 15.2 Morbidity rates of communicable diseases in Romania in 2008 (per 100,000 inhabitants)

Disease	Morbidity rate
Acute diarrheal diseases	342.0
Tuberculosis	87.3
Syphilis	18.7
Viral hepatitis A	14.7
Viral hepatitis B	3.4
Other viral hepatitis	3.6

The specific morbidity rates of communicable diseases are shown in Table 15.2. Tuberculosis remains one of the main concerns, with about 20,000 new cases each year and an increasing percentage of multidrug-resistant cases [3].

15.3 The National System for Emergency Situations Management

The national system for emergency situations management is organized in order to prevent and to manage emergency situations, providing and coordinating human, material, financial, and other resources. Its goal is to keep or to restore the normal status of life and society. The system is organized by the national public administration and consists of a network of bodies and structures with responsibilities in emergency situations management, organized in levels and areas of competence, which have the necessary resources in order to fulfill their legal duties. The main objectives and principles of emergency management are:

- Prediction and prevention,
- Saving people's lives,
- Respect for human rights and freedoms,
- Cooperation on a national and international level,
- Continuity from local authorities to the central public administration, and
- Efficiency, active cooperation, and hierarchy in decision-making.

During emergency situations or potential status of emergency, specific measures are taken in accordance with the legal framework:

- Warning people and institutions of all risks,
- Declaring the state of an imminent threat,
- Preventive and protective measures against a specific risk and, if needed, the decision of total or partial evacuation of the affected area,
- Operative intervention forces and resources available in order to limit or eliminate negative effects,
- Emergency aid,

- Declaring the state of emergency according to conditions stipulated in Article 93 of the Romanian Constitution, and
- Requesting or providing international assistance.

The main components of the National System for Emergency Situations Management are:

- National Committee for Emergency Situations,
- General Inspectorate for Emergency Situations,
- Ministerial emergency committees,
- County and local committees for emergencies, and
- Operational centres for emergency situations.

The National Committee for Emergency Situations is acting under the authority of the Minister of Administration and Interior. When needed, it may be coordinated by the Prime Minister. An Interministerial Committee manages the ordinary activities, which is a body composed of decision makers and experts appointed by the ministries with responsibilities in managing emergencies. A Government Decision from 2004 established the organization and functioning of the National Committee [4]. The Minister of Administration and Interior is the Chairman of the National Committee for Emergency Situations, and a Secretary of State from the same Ministry is the Vice-Chairman. The members are secretaries of state from each ministry or a deputy head of each central public institution. Consultants are also included and they are experts from each ministry and central public institution. The Permanent Technical Secretariat of the National Committee for Emergency Situations functions as a specialized department within the National Operational Centre of the General Inspectorate for Emergency.

The General Inspectorate for Emergency Situations is a specialized department within the Ministry of Administration and Interior, which ensures coordination of activities for prevention and management of emergency situations. The Operational Center of the General Inspectorate is a technical body responsible for evaluation, notification, early warning and operational coordination of national level emergencies. It also ensures functioning of the Permanent Technical Secretariat of the National Committee for Emergency Situations.

The General Inspectorate coordinates and controls specialized public services in emergency situations, ensures cooperation with national civil protection, and is responsible for defence against fire and other emergency situations.

Ministerial emergency committees are established by Ministers or the heads of central public institutions and include decision makers and experts from the ministries and subordinate agencies, with responsibilities in specific emergency management activities. The Ministry of Health has its own committee able to respond and to mobilize resources for public health threats. The composition of a ministerial committee may include representatives of other ministries and institutions involved in the same area of activities.

A county committee for emergencies may be organized under the Prefect, the local representative of the government. The County Committee Board includes heads of decentralized services, local institution managers carrying out functions of county interest, and managers of relevant economic agents. The organization, powers and operational tasks of county committees are established by the decision of the Prefect. In the cities, towns, district of Bucharest, and other administrative divisions, local emergency committees may be established. A local committee is coordinated by a mayor and includes representatives of key public services and institutions from the administrative territory. The organization, powers, and functioning of local committees are established by decision of the mayor, endorsed by the prefect of the county.

15.4 Romanian System of Surveillance and Control of Communicable Diseases

The Ministry of Health (MoH) is responsible for all public health issues, including communicable diseases. The National Institute of Public Health (NIPH) was established in 2009 under the authority of the MoH [5]. Together with the National Institute of Research and Development in Microbiology and Immunology "Cantacuzino" and the National Institute for Infectious Diseases "Prof. Dr. Matei Bals", it coordinates the surveillance and control of communicable diseases, early warning and response to health threats, the public health microbiological laboratory capacities, and preventive measures that should be taken in case of epidemics.

15.4.1 Short History

In 2001, the MoH decided to assess the capacity of early warning and response in order to better control communicable diseases. For this purpose it received technical assistance from the WHO/Regional Office for Europe, and a team of Romanian and international specialists made a comprehensive assessment of the institutional, technical and legislative situation and capacities. In order to improve the existing situation and to develop a surveillance system compatible with the EU, the MoH accepted the recommendations made by the WHO/Europe team. The opportunity to develop the surveillance system came with an EU-sponsored PHARE project "Improving the Romanian System for Epidemiological Surveillance and Control of Communicable Diseases" that lasted from early 2003 until October 2004. The beneficiaries and participants involved in the PHARE project were the MoH through the Department of Public Health, the four regional public health institutes (Bucharest, Cluj, Iasi, Timisoara) and also the 42 district public health directorates and the National Institute for Research and Development in Microbiology and Immunology "Cantacuzino" through its national reference laboratories [1]. Two other institutions with responsibilities for specific surveillance networks are the National Institute for Infectious Diseases "Prof. Dr. Matei Bals" for HIV/AIDS and the Institute for Pneumology "Marius Nasta" for tuberculosis, but they did not directly participate in the PHARE project.

The recommendations made by the international expert team involved in the PHARE project were taken into account in developing a national action plan for the improvement of the communicable disease surveillance system in Romania. The main point was to establish a national competent body, which should be able to:

- Be responsible for the funding and performance management of the regional and district public health structures;
- Maintain consolidated national health surveillance databases for communicable diseases;
- Use surveillance data for the development, publication and dissemination of national policies and good practices in the field of public health;
- Represent the interests of the MoH, in respect of training in the field of communicable diseases, with all national training bodies (undergraduate and postgraduate);
- Represent Romania in all specialist public health functions related to communicable diseases necessary for international cooperation and legal purposes.

The MoH, through Order 123/2003, approved the national action plan. Based on those recommendations, a National Centre for Communicable Diseases Surveillance and Control (NCCDSC) was established. This centre became operational in January 2005. It was located in the Institute of Public Health Bucharest, with the main objective to coordinate the whole national communicable diseases network. Other roles mentioned in the national action plan included monitoring of the national immunization programmes, coordinating the system of early warning and rapid response at the national level, and the management of a dedicated information system.

15.4.2 Current Situation

At present, the NIPH is a coordinating body of a communicable diseases network (Fig. 15.1), through the NCCDSC. NIPH is a body designated to represent the Romanian Government for the purposes set out in the EU decisions 2119/98/EC, 2000/57/EC and all subsequent amendments, and in the reporting functions designated in 2003/542/EC. Recently, NIPH has been designated an ECDC Coordinating Competent Body. Main tasks of the NIPH are:

- Coordination of the national surveillance and control of communicable diseases network;
- Technical coordination of the national alert system for communicable diseases;
- Technical coordination of the rapid response in case of outbreaks or other public health events;
- Surveillance, response, threat detection and training;
- Monitoring and evaluation of the national immunization programme;
- Coordination of the information system on communicable diseases, reporting to international organizations.

The regional public health institutes are responsible for:

- Coordination of the epidemiological activities of the district public health directorates;

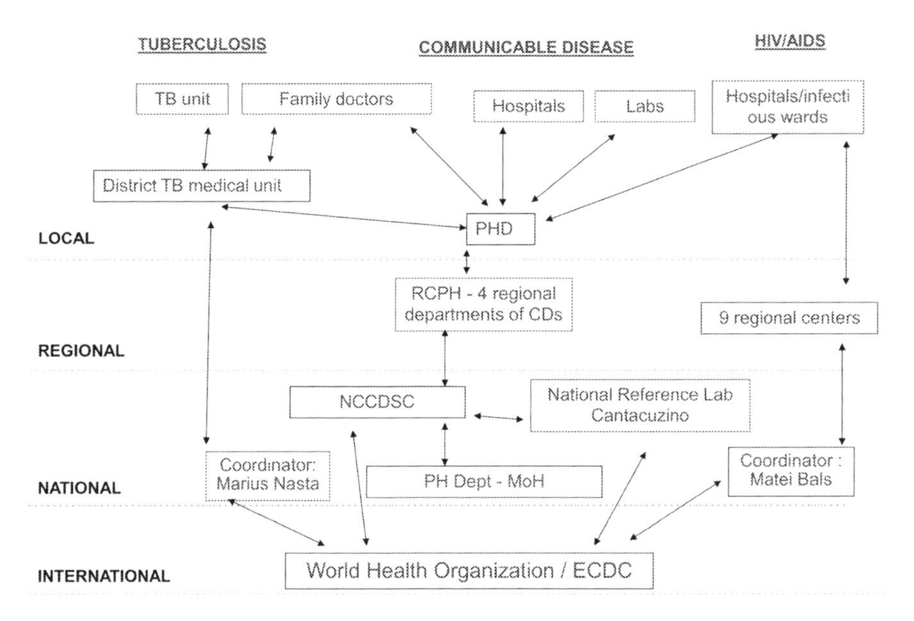

Fig. 15.1 Structure of the communicable diseases network in Romania

- Surveillance and analysis, and coordination of interventions when needed at a regional level;
- Technical assistance to the district public health directorates;
- Diagnosis of communicable diseases, if expert level is needed;
- Training activities in the field of public health.

The district public health directorates are subordinated to the NCCDSC and the regional public health institutes. The district public health directorates:

- Collect data from the existing sources within the territory and analyze communicable diseases data based on time, place, person, and trend for early warning and rapid response;
- Participate in risk assessments for events threatening public health and having a potential national and international spread, organize and administer local communicable diseases databases;
- Report, according to legal regulations, the notifiable communicable diseases;
- Collaborate with NGOs in the process of communicable diseases surveillance;
- Verify how family doctors detect and report cases of communicable diseases;
- Monitor and verify how methodologies and protocols for etiological diagnosis of communicable diseases are implemented;
- Organize epidemiological investigations, identify and coordinate the required measures in order to limit outbreaks of communicable diseases in communities;
- Develop specific activities within the framework of emergency intervention plans.

Infectious disease hospitals report HIV/AIDS data to the eight regional HIV centres (Bucharest, Brasov, Cluj, Timisoara, Craiova, Constanta, Iasi, and Targu-Mures). These centres then report to the national level at the Institute for Infectious Diseases, where data are processed in the HIV/AIDS Monitoring and Evaluation Department. At the district level, forms are also sent to the district public health directorates, which also gather information on HIV testing activities in blood centres and laboratories.

For tuberculosis, suspected cases are diagnosed and confirmed by the tuberculosis district hospital. Both family physicians and tuberculosis specialists from the nearest tuberculosis centre are responsible for case notification and for completing the case management form. The completed form is forwarded to the district tuberculosis dispensary, and from there to the district health statistics office and to the national level at the Institute of Pneumology.

15.5 Public Health Microbiological Laboratories

The public health network has three levels of microbiological diagnostic activities: national (through the national reference laboratories), regional, and local. At the national level there is the National Institute for Research and Development in Microbiology and Immunology "Cantacuzino". Established in 1923, the "Cantacuzino" Institute is a well known Romanian medical institution highly specialized in microbiological diagnostics and in vaccine production. Within the Institute, there are three units responsible for public health, vaccine production and R&D. The national reference laboratories were refurbished and equipped through the PHARE and World Bank projects between 2003 and 2005.

There are ten national reference laboratories, some of them with distinct units inside (see Table 15.3). The staff is 120, and 59 are highly qualified (medical doctors, biologists, biochemists). Microbiological diagnostics at the "Cantacuzino" Institute started in 1950 and continued in various organizational formats. Available services for microbiological diagnosis include 107 usual tests, 39 serology tests, and 53 highly specialized diagnostic procedures. A BSL-3 laboratory is under development through a World Bank project [6].

The number of tests performed by national reference laboratories is around 40,000 per year, but the estimated capacities are at least three times higher, 125,000 per year being a reasonable work load. The problem regarding the relative small number of tests performed, especially those regarding the circulation of microbial strains in Romania, is linked to the financing model of the "Cantacuzino" Institute which is not a state budget institution and needs to have dedicated contracts with regional and local public health authorities in order to perform microbiological investigations. This subject is under discussion and a direct financing from the state budget should be implemented.

The quality of work done by the national reference laboratories is certified by External Quality Assessment (EQA) schemes for many of the microbiological diagnostic procedures performed: polio, influenza, measles, HIV, diphtheria,

Table 15.3 The structure of the national reference laboratories in Romania

	National reference laboratory	Units
1	Viral respiratory transmitted diseases	Influenza, measles, mumps, respiratory syncytial virus
2	Bacterial respiratory transmitted diseases	*Streptococcus, Meningococcus, Haemophilus, Bordetella pertussis, Corynebacterium diphtheriae*
3	Viral food borne diseases	Enterovirus
4	Bacterial food borne diseases	*Salmonella*, other G negative *Shigella, E. coli, Vibrio*
5	Sexually transmitted diseases and blood transmitted diseases	HIV, *Treponema, Neisseria gonorrhoeae, Chlamydia* and *Mycoplasma*
6	Vector borne diseases and entomology	*Rickettsia, Borrelia,* Arbovirus
7	Zoonoses and anaerobic infections	*Bacillus anthracis, Brucella, Listeria, Leptospira*
8	Nosocomial infections and antimicrobial resistance	*Staphylococcus, Pseudomonas,* other G negative non-fermenters, fungi
9	Parasitic infections	
10	Molecular epidemiology	

Salmonella and other gram-negatives, gram-positives, parasitology, antibiotic susceptibility testing, and *Legionella, Borrelia* and pertussis.

Many public health diagnostic activities were performed, and all important epidemiological threats were controlled by the national reference laboratories. Among these threats were West Nile Virus epidemics in 1996 and 2010, anthrax suspect samples (hundreds of tests performed in 2001 and 2002), SARS in 2003, measles in 2005, avian influenza in 2006, H1N1 influenza pandemic in 2009.

The "Cantacuzino" Institute is a member of various WHO and ECDC networks:

- WHO: FLUNET (Influenza Surveillance Network), Global Polio Eradication Initiative;
- ECDC: EVD (emerging and vector borne diseases), VPD (vaccine preventable diseases), FWD (food and water borne diseases), AMR (antimicrobial resistance), HAI (healthcare associated infections), influenza, invasive bacterial infections, zoonoses;
- Research/public health networks: FLUSECURE, REVERSE.

The "Cantacuzino" Institute is also a member of the Pasteur and Associated Institutes Network, many of its specialists having been trained in this network, beginning in 1991. Other roles of the "Cantacuzino" Institute include: national bacterial strains collection, reference material source, and scientific advisor for the MoH and other interested stakeholders. Specialists from the "Cantacuzino" Institute represent Romania in different international technical bodies at the UN, WHO, and ECDC.

The regional centres for public health in Cluj, Iasi, and Timisoara have important microbiological laboratory capacities in terms of staff and equipment, and are responsible for complex diagnostics of communicable diseases in their catchment areas. The "Cantacuzino" Institute is functioning also as a regional centre for the southern part of Romania.

Local district public health directorates have various microbiological laboratory facilities. Some of them, and especially those located at medical universities, are well equipped and have trained personnel. Others use the resources of the regional public health institutes and perform only basic tests themselves.

15.6 National Network for Treatment of Communicable Diseases

The National Institute for Infectious Diseases "Prof. Dr. Matei Bals" is a coordinating body of a network of nine regional centres for the treatment of communicable diseases. The centres were developed in 2007, after the threat of avian flu epidemics. The network is part of a World Bank project which financed necessary investments for care and treatment facilities, including intensive care units, microbiological laboratory equipment, and other logistic needs.

At present, the network is functional and some locations were tested during the H1N1 influenza pandemic that also affected Romania, when hundreds of patients were hospitalized and treated, especially in the central unit, the National Institute for Infectious Diseases "Prof. Dr. Matei Bals".

The network was developed based on the existing one for surveillance and treatment of HIV/AIDS. After 1990, Romania registered an important number of HIV/AIDS cases, affecting especially children. This situation required extraordinary measures, and one of them was to organize a medical network able to treat and to offer counseling and preventive measures to affected people. This network, coordinated by the National Institute for Infectious Diseases "Prof. Dr. Matei Bals", is hosting the database of HIV/AIDS infected people and has achieved important results in the control of the disease [5]. The Romanian government has given significant financial resources and HAART therapy is offered to more than 8,000 patients.

The Institute of Pneumology "Marius Nasta" has similar responsibilities regarding surveillance and treatment of tuberculosis infections. At the local level many facilities (hospitals, laboratories) are dedicated to these patients. Tuberculosis represents one of the main challenges for the public health system in Romania, with more than 20,000 new cases each year, important national and international (Global Fund) resources being allotted.

Both institutes are working together with NCCDSC. Epidemiological data from the local level for HIV/AIDS and tuberculosis are sent periodically to district public health directorates and to NCCDSC.

15.7 Surveillance of Communicable Diseases

The communicable diseases surveillance network is financed by the state budget under the National Programme on Community Health. Treatment of communicable diseases is covered by the public health insurance funds.

The reporting system covers 65 communicable diseases. These are classified as: (1) Diseases with nominal immediate notification by phone; (2) Diseases with nominal notification within 24 h after detection; and (3) Diseases with numerical periodic reporting (weekly, monthly, quarterly, and annually). Detection and notification of communicable diseases are among the responsibilities of family doctors, of ambulatory units and of hospitals, mainly of the infectious diseases hospitals, or other specialized units [7].

The confirmation of cases is done in districts and in Bucharest by the laboratories of the local district public health directorate, and/or by the regional and national reference laboratories. The transmission of data is by phone or by fax, and the notification forms for each communicable disease case are sent by mail or courier service. Data analysis is carried out in a few districts at the local level; usually data analysis is conducted at regional and national levels and the feedback to the district is limited. The surveillance of certain communicable diseases (tuberculosis, HIV/AIDS) is done also in parallel systems using a separate informational flow.

A group of 11 communicable diseases – wild polio virus infection, influenza with a new virus subtype, cholera, plague, hemorrhagic fevers, yellow fever, smallpox, varioloid, SARS, an unexpected infectious disease, and an unexpected health event – are reported immediately; the district public health directorates report immediately to the Bureau for International Health Regulation and Toxicology Information (BIHRTI), an office within the National Institute of Public Health (which is the focal point for IHR). NCCDSC verifies the information and together with BIHRTI informs the MoH which notifies the WHO. These cases have to be confirmed by national reference laboratories [7].

Another group of 25 communicable diseases has to be reported immediately by phone to the district public health directorates by all medical assistance providers. Within 24 h, the district public health directorate sends the report to the regional public health institute. Further reports are sent to the NCCDSC and BIHRTI, which inform the MoH, after evaluating the level of importance for the epidemiological event. Written forms are also sent to the authorities mentioned.

There are ten communicable diseases which are reported on a monthly basis to the district public health directorates by all the medical assistance providers. Aggregated data on influenza, acute respiratory infections, acute diarrheal disease, West Nile meningo-encephalitis, and other communicable diseases are reported on weekly basis, using specific methodologies.

For all communicable diseases the medical assistance providers send to the district public health directorates a notification form 5 days after detection. District public health directorates send the duplicates of the notification forms to the regional public health institutes, which send the regional data to NCCDSC.

NCCDSC, the competent body for communicable diseases surveillance, reports to ECDC the diseases under 2119/98/EC Decision, after the validation of cases. The regional public health institutes provide quarterly and annual reports for the regions. NCCDSC and BIHRTI also provide quarterly and annual reports, which are sent to the MoH.

Table 15.4 Confirmed and suspect cases of communicable diseases of bioterrorism concern in Romania in 2010

Disease	Number of confirmed cases	Number of suspect cases reported	Percentage of confirmation
Malaria	19	20	95
Viral hemorrhagic fever (Hantavirus)	4	10	40
Typhoid fever	3	4	75
Botulism	23	29	79.3
Tetanus	9	12	75
Avian flu	–	–	–
Anthrax	–	3	–

15.8 Early Warning System

In 2005, the Minister of Health ordered the methodology for early warning and rapid response. The list of communicable diseases included in this system are smallpox, plague, acute hemorrhagic fevers, SARS, syndromes that could raise the suspicion of a communicable disease: acute watery diarrhea for cholera suspicion, acute diarrhea with or without blood, acute icteric syndrome, acute infections of the lower respiratory tract, rubella suspicion, meningitis/encephalitis suspicion, malaria suspicion, fever of unknown origin and unknown disease occurring in a cluster. The methodology is based on case definitions, alert thresholds, defining responsibilities and information flow, and providing the reporting format [7].

Family doctors detect, notify and report the case and transfer the patient to the specialist for infectious diseases, who notifies by phone the event and fills a dedicated warning report submitted to the district public health directorate.

The infectious diseases hospital confirms or invalidates the suspicion and notifies the district public health directorate, which, through its epidemiology unit, analyses data from health care providers and takes the measures of active detection of cases and control and sends a preliminary report of epidemiological warning to the regional public health institute, and further on to NCCDSC. Diagnosis is confirmed by national reference laboratories.

Local measures are taken by district public health directorates, with technical assistance from the regional level. If the outbreak is spreading and affects more than one region the NCCDSC takes the lead and organizes measures, reporting to the MoH and to the international organizations.

Table 15.4 presents the list of confirmed and suspect cases of communicable diseases in 2010 which represent a main threat for public health and are of bioterrorism concern [3]. Until now, no evidence of bioterrorism has been registered in Romania.

15.9 Conclusions

The capacity of the Romanian authorities to respond to different health threats due to communicable diseases has improved in the last few years in terms of diagnostic capacities and organizational matters. Early warning and efficiency of response of the epidemiological surveillance system was proven during the H1N1 influenza pandemic and in other communicable diseases emergencies.

The improvements registered in the last few years include data collection and reporting methodology for communicable diseases surveillance, information flow of the unique notification form for communicable diseases, and establishment of the National Electronic Register for Communicable Diseases.

The district public health authorities are the focal point for all the communicable diseases notified in the district and data are validated at the regional and national level.

The main threats are represented by emerging and re-emerging communicable diseases due to intensified international traffic of persons and goods and bioterrorist events.

From an organizational point of view, education of family doctors should improve their capability to recognize and report communicable diseases and apply control measures at the source. Elaboration of the national surveillance manual is needed as well as enhancing the laboratory capacities and implementing a reliable information system for communicable diseases based on a new technological platform.

Strengthening cooperation with emergency staff from the Ministry of Administration and Interior and from other government bodies responsible for security of social and economic activities is desired.

References and Further Reading

1. Stevens R (2004) Final report to delegation of EC in Bucharest regarding PHARE project, EuropeAid/113121/D/SV/RO, technical assistance for improving the Romanian system for epidemiological surveillance and control of communicable diseases, Bucharest
2. The Dubrovnik pledge on surveillance and prioritization of infectious diseases – report on a WHO meeting, Bucharest, Romania, 21–23 Nov 2002
3. National Institute of Public Health Bucharest (2011) Report on communicable diseases 2009, report of NCCDSC activity, 2011, www.insp.gov.ro
4. General inspectorate for emergency situations (Government Decisions 1489, 1490/2004, 1514/2005)
5. Vladescu C, Scîntee G, Olsavszky V, Allin S, Mladovsky P (2008) Romania: health system review. Health systems in transition 10(3):1–172
6. Ionescu G, Codita I, Canton A (2010) Role of the microbiology NRLs in the European context, updated presentation on 23rd meeting of the ECDC advisory forum, 29–30 Sept 2010

Chapter 16
Case Study – Serbia

Goran Belojevic

Abstract Recent turbulent historic events in the territory of Serbia have been an enormous challenge for the Serbian Government and disaster responders in coping with war destruction, the problem of hundreds of thousands of refugees and internally displaced persons and usual natural disasters. Furthermore, the geographic position on the crossroads between East and West and North and South and the relatively unstable political situation and disputed status of the Kosovo territory actualizes the possibility of terrorism, including bioterrorism, as a method of fulfilling political aims. Serbia's public health system is largely based on the principles from the former Yugoslavia, but it needs further improvement to successfully cope with a bioterrorism threat. At the moment there is a gap between a non-favourable political and security position of Serbia and its public health preparedness for bioterrorism.

16.1 Introduction

Organized disaster management in Serbia started with the establishment of the Serbian Society of the Red Cross in 1876 [11]. In the Kingdom of Yugoslavia the state was involved for the first time in disaster management in 1932 with the publication of "the General Instructions for the Work for the Protection of the Country in Case of the Enemy Attack from the Air". The Yugoslav Ministry of the Army and Navy organized regional headquarters that were responsible for public information, first aid, and evacuation in the case of bombing [2].

G. Belojevic (✉)
Institute of Hygiene and Medical Ecology, Faculty of Medicine, University of Belgrade, Belgrade, Serbia
e-mail: goran.belojevic@hotmail.com

I. Hunger et al. (eds.), *Biopreparedness and Public Health: Exploring Synergies*, NATO Science for Peace and Security Series A: Chemistry and Biology,
DOI 10.1007/978-94-007-5273-3_16,

After World War II, in the People's Republic of Yugoslavia, the Ministry of Interior joined the Army in protecting the citizens from air raids by adopting the "Regulation on Organization and Work of the Division for Anti-Aircraft Protection" [8]. After introducing the Law on People's Defence in 1955, the Civil Protection Service replaced the Division for Anti-Aircraft Protection in the Ministry of Interior with wide responsibilities in all kinds of disasters. From 1963, the Armed Forces, the Civil Protection Service, and the Monitoring and Alert Service were integral parts of the Ministry of Defence. The Civil Protection System was organized through municipal units and headquarters with experts and the equipment for the protection and rescue of people in disasters [4]. After introducing the Law on Emergency Situations in 2009 [6], the Ministry of Interior of Serbia returned to the position of the main state organization for the strategy and planning of civil protection and rescue in disasters. In the event of a national disaster, the President will order the Chief of the General Staff to mobilize the Army. In the case of emergency on the whole territory of Serbia the Government forms the Republic Headquarters for Emergency Situation and the regional headquarters.

In 2002, the Ministry of Interior established the Department of Protection and Rescue, responsible for coordinating the response to all kinds of disasters. Of its 3,000 officers, 150 are prevention inspectors and the remainder are firemen. Police and gendarmerie are engaged to provide security at the local level. At the municipal level, the mayor is responsible for establishing a crisis headquarter staffed by the appropriate experts. The Department of Civil Protection within the Ministry of Defence authorizes civil protection officers at the municipal level as expert advisors to the crisis committee. They communicate with both the military and civilian disaster responders and typically have four to five staff and basic equipment for protection and rescue.

In 2007, the Army created a specialized department dedicated to civil-military cooperation. Organizational subunits have been designated for this purpose with the primary function to communicate and coordinate with other non-military crisis responders.

The system of civil protection and rescue in disasters is funded from the Republic Budget, the budget of local communities and from the special Fund for Emergency Situations.

16.2 Recent Disasters in Serbia

War conflicts in Croatia and Bosnia and Herzegovina in the 1990s brought hundreds of thousands of refugees into Serbia as an unbearable burden for the country exhausted by the UN sanctions imposed in 1992. Unrest in Kosovo and subsequent NATO bombing made the situation much more difficult for Serbia. In 2001, there were 450,000 internally displaced people [3]. In the first decade of the twenty-first century, besides the refugee problem, the Serbian Government had to face usual disasters such as landslides, floods, forest fires, and transportation accidents. In managing refugee and disaster problems the government engaged police, civil protection, the Army, the Red Cross of Serbia, the Ministry of Agriculture, Forestry, and Water, the Ministry of Environment, the Ministry of Energy, Border Police and the Veterinary Agency.

16.3 Public Health System and Health Indicators in Serbia

The area of the Republic of Serbia is 88,361 sq km (77,474 sq km excluding Kosovo) and the population is around 10.1 million (around 7.3 million excluding Kosovo). Population density is 114 individuals per sq km (94 individuals per sq km excluding Kosovo).

Public health care in Serbia is organized through the network of state and private health institutions. There is a network of 23 public health institutes with the Republic Public Health Institute "Milan Jovanovic-Batut" as a coordinating institution. Furthermore, there are 159 health care centres, 37 general hospitals, 14 specialised hospitals, and 5 university clinical centres. In the private sector there are 1,220 medical offices and clinics, 149 laboratories, 81 hospitals and 58 polyclinics.

The Global Health Observatory for Serbia [15] reported that life expectancy at birth in 2008 was 71 years for males and 76 years for females. The adult mortality rate per 1,000 people aged 15–59 years is 138, lower than the Balkan region average of 149. Under-five mortality rate per 1,000 live births is 8, lower than the Balkan region average of 14. Total expenditure for health in Serbia is 8.2% of GDP, close to the 8.9% average expenditure in the OECD countries. However, health expenditure per capita is 4.7 times lower than the average expenditure in the EU, 525 and 2,468 USD, respectively. Comparing other indicators of health care in Serbia and Europe there is also a worse situation in Serbia: physicians per 1,000 people – 2.01 and 3.25, respectively; nurses and midwives per 1,000 people – 4.43 and 6.81, respectively; beds per 1,000 people – 5.57 and 7.60, respectively.

16.4 Major Infectious Diseases in Serbia

According to the Serbian Law on Population Protection from Infectious Diseases [5], there are 70 infectious diseases with regular measures of registration and protection:

1. Cholera	36. Creutzfeldt–Jakob disease
2. Typhoid fever	37. Rabies-lyssa
3. Other salmonelloses	38. Tick borne viral encephalitis
4. Shigellosis	39. Enteroviral meningitis
5. Campylobacter enteritis	40. Yellow fever
6. Yersinia enterocolitica enteritis	41. Lassa fever
7. Other bacterial intestinal infections	42. Crimean-Congo fever
8. Staphylococcal food intoxication	43. Marburg hemorrhagic fever
9. Botulism	44. Ebola hemorrhagic fever
10. Other bacterial food poisoning	45. Hantavirus hemorrhagic fever with renal syndrome
11. Amebiasis	46. Chickenpox
12. Lambliasis	47. Smallpox
13. Cryptosporidiosis	48. Morbilli
14. Infectious diarrhea and gastroenteritis	49. Rubeola
15. Tuberculosis	50. Congenital rubeola syndrome
16. Plague	51. Acute hepatitis A
17. Tularemia	52. Acute hepatitis B
18. Anthrax	53. Acute hepatitis C
19. Brucellosis	54. Acute hepatitis E
20. Leptospirosis	55. Chronic hepatitis B,C
21. Listeriosis	56. Unspecified viral hepatitis
22. Tetanus	57. AIDS
23. Diphtheria	58. Parotitis
24. Pertussis	59. Infectious mononucleosis
25. Scarlet fever	60. Malaria
26. Meningococcal infection	61. Leishmaniasis
27. Septicemia	62. Toxoplasmosis
28. Legionellosis	63. Echinococcosis
29. Syphilis	64. Trichinellosis
30. Gonococcal infection	65. Scabies
31. Chlamydia sexually transmitted disease	66. Haemophilus influenza
32. Lyme disease	67. Bacterial meningitis
33. Psittacosis	68. Streptococcal pharyngitis and tonsillitis
34. Q fever	69. Influenza
35. Poliomyelitis	70. Viral and bacterial pneumonia.

During 2009, there were 431,666 cases of infectious diseases in Serbia, which is a 22% increase compared to the year 2008. This is the largest number of cases of infectious diseases in the period 2005–2009 after an increasing 5-year trend (Fig. 16.1). This increase is mainly due to the 2009 pandemic influenza outbreak and other respiratory infections.

The most common infectious diseases in Serbia according to the incidence rate during 2005–2009, were: (1) streptococcal pharyngitis, (2) streptococcal tonsillitis, (3) chickenpox, (4) influenza, (5) pneumonia, (6) infectious diarrheal diseases, (7) other bacterial intestinal infections, (8) scabies, (9) scarlet fever, (10) mononucleosis,

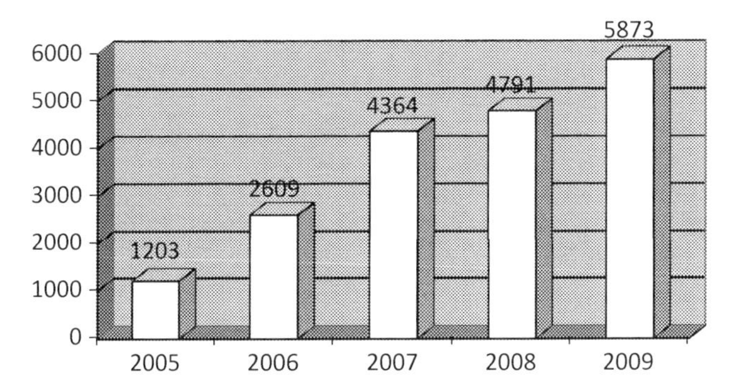

Fig. 16.1 Incidence of infectious diseases (per 100,000 inhabitants) in Serbia, 2005–2009 (Source: Knezevic T (ed) (2009), Health Statistical Yearbook of the Republic of Serbia, Institute of Public Health "Dr Milan Jovanovic-Batut", Belgrade: Elit medica)

(11) bacterial food poisoning, (12) salmonellosis, (13) Chlamydia sexually transmitted disease, (14) tuberculosis, and (15) Lyme disease (Table 16.1).

In 2009, there were 245 lethal cases from infectious diseases, mostly from pandemic influenza. This is the largest mortality rate from infectious diseases in the period 2005–2009 (Fig. 16.2). Other leading causes of mortality from infectious diseases in Serbia in the period 2005–2009 are tuberculosis, sepsis, AIDS, pneumonia, and meningitis (Table 16.2).

16.5 Infectious Diseases as a Potential Bioterrorism Threat in Serbia

Concerning the infectious diseases that might be perceived as a potential bioterrorism threat, the outbreak of smallpox in Yugoslavia in 1972 was the last major outbreak of smallpox in Europe. It was centered in Kosovo and Belgrade. The epidemic was started by a Muslim pilgrim upon returning from the Middle East to Kosovo. There were 175 infected people, 35 of whom died. The epidemic lasted 3 months and was efficiently contained by enforced quarantine and mass vaccination. Although the WHO declared smallpox fully eradicated in 1980, the possibility of future bioterrorism attacks, which may cause a new outbreak of smallpox and return smallpox into Serbia is perceived as serious, due to the unstable political situation in Serbia and the unresolved Kosovo problem [10]. Among other diseases from the Category A potential bioterrorist agents the largest number of cases in the period 2005–2009 was from tularemia. However, no possibility of deliberate epidemics of anthrax, botulism, and tularemia were investigated during this period (Table 16.3).

The specific circumstances of the early post-war period in Kosovo in 1999 and 2000 and a large outbreak of tularemia with 327 cases in 21 of 29 Kosovo municipalities were the reasons for engagement of a WHO team to investigate the

Table 16.1 The most common infectious diseases in Serbia, 2005–2009 (incidence rate per 100,000 inhabitants (rank)) (Source: Knezevic T (ed.) Health Statistical Yearbooks of the Republic of Serbia 2005–2009, Institute of Public Health "Dr Milan Jovanovic-Batut", Belgrade: Elit medica)

Disease	2005	2006	2007	2008	2009
Streptococcal pharyngitis	21 (11)	580 (2)	1165 (1)	1492 (1)	1941 (1)
Streptococcal tonsillitis	101 (2)	604 (1)	922 (2)	927 (3)	1143 (2)
Influenza	16 (12)	124 (6)	756 (3)	936 (2)	1604 (3)
Chickenpox	529 (1)	513 (3)	664 (4)	582 (4)	498 (4)
Pneumonia	46 (6)	174 (4)	227 (5)	250 (5)	212 (5)
Infectious diarrheal diseases	82 (3)	159 (5)	135 (6)	173 (6)	117 (6)
Scabies	48 (5)	61 (8)	65 (8)	59 (8)	54 (7)
Other bacterial intestinal infections	80 (4)	90 (7)	69 (7)	72 (7)	52 (8)
Scarlet fever	34 (8)	43 (9)	53 (9)	36 (9)	33 (9)
Tuberculosis	4 (14)	30 (13)	27 (13)	24 (13)	32 (10)
Mononucleosis	26 (9)	29 (14)	35 (10)	36 (10)	32 (11)
Salmonellosis	29 (10)	31 (12)	35 (11)	23 (14)	27 (12)
Chlamydia sexually transmitted disease	2 (15)	40 (11)	15 (14)	32 (11)	27 (13)
Bacterial food poisoning	46 (7)	42 (10)	32 (12)	31 (12)	20 (14)
Lyme disease	6 (13)	7 (15)	9 (15)	12 (15)	13 (15)

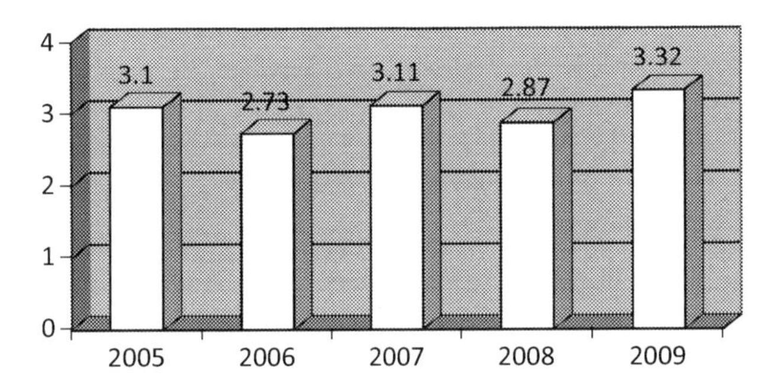

Fig. 16.2 Mortality rate (per 100,000 inhabitants) from infectious diseases in Serbia, 2005–2009 (Source: Knezevic T (ed) (2009), Health Statistical Yearbook of the Republic of Serbia, Institute of Public Health "Dr Milan Jovanovic-Batut", Belgrade: Elit medica)

possibility of a deliberate epidemic. Matched analysis of 46 case households and 76 control households suggested that infection was transmitted through contaminated food or water and that the source of infection was rodents. Environmental circumstances in war-torn Kosovo led to an epizootic rodent tularemia and its spread to resettled rural populations living under circumstances of sub-standard housing, hygiene, and sanitation. Analysis of cases showed no unexpected fulminant course of the disease, response to usual therapy, no unusual coexisting syndromes, and no

Table 16.2 The leading causes of death from infectious diseases in Serbia, 2005–2009 (number/mortality rate per 100,000 inhabitants/rank) [9]

Disease	2005	2006	2007	2008	2009
Influenza	1/0.01/-	0	1/0.01/-	0	52/0.71/1
Tuberculosis	61/0.79/2	55/0.73/2	69/0.93/1	53/0.72/1	51/0.69/2
Sepsis	67/0.89/1	59/0.78/1	46/0.62/2/3	50/0.68/2	48/0.65/3
AIDS	26/0.33/3	24/0.32/3	15/0.20/5	22/0.29/4	25/0.34/4
Pneumonia	19/0.25/4	21/0.27/4/5	46/0.62/2/3	31/0.42/3	22/0.30/5
Meningitis	14/0.18/5	20/0.27/4/5	24/0.32/4	21/0.28/5	20/0.27/6

Table 16.3 Number of cases and incidence rate per 100,000 inhabitants in Serbia of infectious diseases from the Category A of potential bioterrorist agents, 2005–2009 [9]

Disease	2005	2006	2007	2008	2009
Cutaneous anthrax	1 (0.01)	0	0	4 (0.05)	1 (0.01)
Botulism	10 (0.13)	6 (0.08)	19 (0.26)	4 (0.05)	7 (0.10)
Tularemia	56 (0.74)	36 (0.48)	7 (0.09)	25 (0.34)	2 (0.03)

human deaths. Concerning geographic and seasonal distribution, the disease was endemic in the area, with a usual geographic distribution, and with a typical seasonal distribution with the peak in January 2000, and with no simultaneous occurrences of cases that could have mimicked a biological attack. The pathogen was permanently present in the region with smaller or larger epidemics during former decades in the area. The epidemic was not explosive. The provided evidence supported the conclusion that this epidemic of tularemia was a natural event, most likely resulting from unusual environmental and socio-political circumstances in war-torn Kosovo [7, 12].

According to the Law on population protection from infectious diseases (2003–2004) in the case of epidemics of plague, smallpox and viral hemorrhagic fever (Ebola, Marburg, Crimean-Congo, Lassa) mandatory isolation of patients and quarantine of persons who were in contact with diseased are ordered by the Minister of Health. Persons who come from the countries with cases of cholera, plague, smallpox, yellow fever and hemorrhagic fever and malaria are under health surveillance. These persons have to report regularly to an authorized Public Health Institute for a medical check-up. In the case of a possible bioterrorist attack the Minister of Health declares an epidemic of a major epidemiological importance and orders the anti-epidemic measures and epidemiologic surveillance.

Concerning bioterrorism preparedness in Serbia, the main coordinator is the National Institute of Public Health in Belgrade with its Department for Bioterrorism and Crisis Management which is not yet fully staffed. The Institute's Epidemiology Department receives data on the cases of infectious diseases on a bi-weekly basis.

However, a recent external analysis of the preparedness of Serbia for disasters including bioterrorism concludes that the "Ministry of Health and individual hospitals are not adequately engaged in disaster planning", that "if specific protocols do exist, they are not widely known", and that there is "a lack of insight by outside agencies into the plans and protocols of the Ministry" [14].

The most serious terrorist threat in Serbia comes from Wahhabism in the Serbian province of Raska, and from Kosovo. In July 2009, 12 Wahhabis were sentenced to a total of 60 years in jail for preparing terrorist attacks on targets in Belgrade: National Theatre, Beogradjanka Building, Hotel Park, and the US Embassy [13]. In August 2009, the Special Court in Belgrade sentenced four Wahhabis to a total of 27 years in prison. The group was accused of preparing terrorist acts throughout Serbia, including, according to the indictment, a planned attack on a football match in Novi Pazar [1].

16.6 Conclusion

Although Serbia has not faced a bioterrorist attack so far, an unstable political situation, the disputed position of the Kosovo territory, and two recently sentenced Wahhabi terrorist groups support the hypothesis that bioterrorism may also be used in fulfilling political aims. At the moment, the Serbian public health system is not satisfactorily prepared for a bioterrorist attack and organizational improvements are needed.

References

1. B92 News (2009) Wahhabis sentenced to 27 years prison. http://www.b92.net/eng/news/crimes-article. Accessed 30 Apr 2011
2. Djarmati DJ, Jakovljević V (1996) Civil protection in SRJ. Studentski trg, Belgrade (in Serbian)
3. Faculty of Civil Defence (2004) Indicators of human security in Serbia. Faculty of Civil Defence, Belgrade
4. Federal Secretariat for Public Defence (1983) Strategy of armed conflict. Federal Secretariat for Public Defence, Belgrade (in Serbian)
5. Government of Serbia (2003) Law on population protection from infectious diseases (2003–2004), Official Gazette of Serbia (72/2003, 43/2004, 55/2004)
6. Government of Serbia (2009) Law on emergency situations, Official Gazette of Serbia (111/09, 29 December 2009; 92/11, 7 December 2011) (in Serbian)
7. Grunow R, Finke EJ (2002) A procedure for differentiating between the intentional release of biological warfare agents and natural outbreaks of disease: its use in analyzing the tularemia outbreak in Kosovo in 1999 and 2000. Clin Microbiol Infect 8:510–521
8. Jakovljević V (2006) System of civil defence. Faculty of Civil Defence, Belgrade (in Serbian)
9. Knezevic T (ed) (2009) Health Statistical Yearbook of the Republic of Serbia, Institute of Public Health "Dr Milan Jovanovic-Batut". Elit medica, Belgrade
10. Kuljic Kapulica N (2004) Smallpox – in the past or not? Srp Arh Cel Lek 132:272–276

11. Red Cross of Serbia (2011) History. Red Cross of Serbia. http://www.redcross.org.rs. Accessed 26 Apr 2011
12. Reintjes R, Dedushaj I, Gjini A, Jorgensen TR, Cotter B, Lieftucht A, D'Ancona F, Dennis DT, Kosoy MA, Mulliqi-Osmani G, Grunow R, Kalaveshi A, Gashi L, Humolli I (2002) Tularemia outbreak investigation in Kosovo: case control and environmental studies. Emerg Infect Dis 8:69–73
13. Stojanovic D (2009) Serbia sentences Muslims for terrorism. http://www.serbianna.com/news/archives/2624. Accessed 30 Apr 2011
14. Wall E, Chu E, Dimitrijevic I (2008) The civil protection in Serbia. Jefferson Institute, Washington, DC
15. WHO (2011) Global health observatory. Serbia: Country profiles. General health statistical profile. http://www.who.int/gho/countries/srb/country_profiles/en/index.html. Accessed 26 Apr 2011

Chapter 17
Case Study – Turkey

Gurkan Mert

Abstract The use of biological agents in terrorist attacks has focused the world's attention on the development of preparedness and response programmes. The real danger with biological agents, when used as weapons, is their uncontrollable nature. The biological threat differs markedly from the threat posed by chemical or nuclear weapons, forcing changes in terms of research, intelligence gathering, the level of preparedness and the design of response programmes. There are a great number of pathogens that are able to harm human beings, yet only a small subset of them can be labeled potential biowarfare agents. Still, the danger is a very real one and the control of such biological agents requires the coordinated effort of the entire public health community – both civilian and military. There is also a need for a surveillance and notification system across the whole country to detect, identify, and investigate a suspected biological agent and to subsequently implement proper decontamination procedures. This chapter will discuss several specific aspects of the Turkish programme that was established to protect against biological attacks, with a particular focus on the current main public health threats in Turkey (in terms of infectious diseases), the National Notifiable Diseases Surveillance System (NNDSS), the role of the new responsible institution – the Disaster and Emergency Management Presidency (DEMP), the Ministry of Health, Bioterrorism and Preparedness, and medical organizations on the military side.

The views expressed in this paper are those of the author and should not be taken to be a statement of policy of the Turkish Republic.

G. Mert (✉)
Department of Infectious Diseases and Clinical Microbiology,
Gulhane Military Medical Academy, Ankara, Turkey
e-mail: gmert@gata.edu.tr

I. Hunger et al. (eds.), *Biopreparedness and Public Health: Exploring Synergies*,
NATO Science for Peace and Security Series A: Chemistry and Biology,
DOI 10.1007/978-94-007-5273-3_17,

17.1 Introduction

One of the first recorded uses of microorganisms and their toxins as agents of war was in the fourteenth century. In the siege of Kaffa (or Caffa), the Tatar army catapulted corpses infected with plague over the city walls, spreading the disease among the local population. Subsequently, this technique, together with the infecting of sources of drinking water, became a part of warfare and spurred the use of other primitive yet effective techniques. For example, in 1763, blankets contaminated with smallpox virus were delivered to Native American Tribes, and even more recently in Vietnam in the early 1960s, concealed punji sticks tipped with excrement were used to wound and infect US troops [1]. *Bacillus anthracis* was the first bacterium conclusively demonstrated to cause disease and this discovery led to an increased interest in the production of biological agents to be used as a weapon of war. During the Second Sino-Japanese War, biological agents were also used by the Japanese, resulting in the deaths of numerous Chinese [2]. In 1979, 60 people died after being accidentally exposed to anthrax in Sverdlovsk, Russia [7], and more recently, in 2001, letters containing anthrax spores were mailed to several news media offices and two US senators, resulting in the death of five people [4].

The nature of terrorism is changing: it is no longer simply hijackings or bombings. Bioterrorism is not a remote, hypothetical event. On the contrary, a bioterrorist attack has already occurred and could occur again at any time, under any circumstances, and at a magnitude far greater than we have thus far witnessed. Although similar to chemical terrorism in some ways, bioterrorism differs primarily in the lag time between the terrorist event and its medical consequences. It therefore poses its own critical challenges, particularly for the public health community [5].

Several factors make the threat presented by biological weapons unique when compared with chemical and nuclear ones. The use of biological agents in bioterrorism is a tempting choice for the terrorist because biological agents are relatively easy to obtain or produce, can be easily disseminated, and can cause widespread fear and panic beyond the actual physical damage they can cause. Across the world, facilities and equipment that have entirely legitimate, non-threatening applications can be used to produce biological agents. In addition, the low cost of production means that it is relatively easy for poor countries or terrorist organizations to acquire or make them.

Over the past 15 years, there have been advances in biotechnology that could potentially be used in the production of biological agents, including genetically engineered pathogens that are resistant to antimicrobials and classic vaccines. The prospect of an effective bioterrorism attack causing devastation to society is deeply concerning [9].

17.2 Main Public Health Threats in Turkey in Terms of Infectious Diseases

There are several diseases in Turkey that could be used as a biological agent: Crimean Congo hemorrhagic fever, tularemia (with increasing incidence in recent years) and Hanta virus infections (with a very limited number of reported cases).

There is no proof in hand to make us think that they are being used as biological weapons. In fact, the progress of these diseases over the years has shown different characteristics to what would be otherwise expected. For example, the first case of Crimean Congo hemorrhagic fever in Turkey was detected in 2002 and, according to the Turkish Ministry of Health; nearly 322 citizens have lost their lives to it since then. The number of reported deaths from this disease has recently diminished. 1,075 cases were reported in 2011, 54 cases resulted in death. The mortality rate is 5% for Turkey. As a result of the studies carried out by public health bodies, citizens became aware of the disease and may have changed their behavior accordingly. Furthermore, the vaccination of animals against vectors by the Ministry of Agriculture, especially in the regions where plenty of *Hyalomma marginatum* ticks live, has caused the number of cases to come down to manageable levels. RNA analysis revealed that strains in Turkey are similar to strains found in Southwestern Russia, Kosovo and the Balkan.

Crimean Congo hemorrhagic fever and Hanta virus infections are among the viral hemorrhagic diseases that can be produced in cell cultures, but because of insufficient titers their use as a weapon of mass destruction is limited. Another limitation is low stability and requirement of ultra-cold storage conditions [1, 2]. Though Crimean Congo hemorrhagic fever and Hanta virus cases in Turkey at the moment are not perceived as bioterrorism agents, it is thought that the difficulties arising from the possibility of these viruses being used as biological weapons can be overcome through research programmes in the future.

Increased tularemia cases, especially during the summer months in Turkey in recent years, warrant continued attention. Cases are concentrated in the central regions of the country, where drinking water is obtained from wells. Cases are more of the oropharyngeal type and no pulmonary involvement has been reported. The Ministry of Health is responsible for carrying out environmental surveillance and decontamination studies. Response teams are subsequently created and treatment and prophylaxis studies conducted. Diagnosis of the disease is determined through pathology and with the help of reference laboratories certified to at least BSL-2.

17.3 National Notifiable Diseases Surveillance System in Turkey

The Notifiable Diseases Detection and Monitoring of Epidemic Diseases Surveillance System was established in Turkey in order to take the necessary precautions and determine and evaluate any urgent cases of bioterrorism. Through this system, even the most remote provincial agencies responsible for monitoring and recording outbreaks of disease have to report such occurrences to the center. Notification systems are absolutely vital mechanisms for countries to collect data about diseases in a systematic way in order to interpret the frequency of outbreaks and their patterns of behavior, to plan, to predict outbreaks, and to develop and implement programmes to protect and control. The smooth operation of these mechanisms can be primarily achieved through the provision of standards, training, laboratory support, administrative resources, and a robust communications network.

The new notification system is built around "standard case definitions" and infectious disease notification is now based upon evidence derived from the laboratory rather than opinion. With this development, contrary to previous reporting system, a laboratory capable of using valid standard techniques will automatically be included to the system either indirectly (for Group A, B and C diseases) or directly (for Group D diseases) upon diagnosis of the infection.

Group A diseases require the collection of information for notification from all institutions starting from the first level in the health system. In this first step an important proportion of the diseases are ones where notification is triggered by the admission of patients to the first level. Physicians, according to the standard case definition, make the required notification and initiate research. In situations with fewer opportunities for diagnosis, the patient is transferred to the higher level or directly sent to the highest level. In both cases, treatment begins by diagnosing and sending the health information of the patient(s) to the responsible institutions located in the place where each patient lives, via Form 014 to the Provincial Health Directorate and, if a military hospital is involved, to the Turkish Armed Forces Medical Command (TAF MEDCOM). The goal is to find out if similar cases have occurred in the same area to identify the source of the disease.

Group B consists of the diseases whose notification is obligatory according to the 1969 International Health Regulations of World Health Organization (WHO). Although smallpox was eradicated in the late 1970s, it is still on the agenda today because of the potential it has as an agent in biological terrorism. The other diseases in group B are not applicable to Turkey but there are some parts of the world where these diseases still spread with high mortality rates and that is why the continuation of international reporting is necessary. Anybody, regardless of the level they are at when faced with a possible case of any of these diseases, is obliged to notify the Ministry of Health (MoH) and, for military hospitals, the TAF MEDCOM directly and by the fastest means. At the international level, the reporting of these diseases is the sole responsibility of the Health Ministry (Table 17.1).

Group C mostly consists of diseases that have been newly included in the notification system. A common feature of these, except for trachoma, is that notification from the first level is not necessary. Depending on the type of the disease, "sentinel surveillance" is an acceptable way to follow these diseases because:

1. Starting from the second level, some of these diseases can only be identified by more specialized institutions or laboratories, which would then be responsible for notification.
2. In the case of a pandemic influenza outbreak, the rules state that samples from not all cases but from an adequate number of cases should be taken into account, and the fact that this is done at a certain center to control pandemics means that there is an overlap of purpose in achieving the same goal.
3. In some cases, such as Creutzfeldt-Jakob disease (CJD) or congenital rubella, the return of information to the first level and the notification of the information

Table. 17.1 List of the 51 infectious diseases and pathogens that constitute groups A, B, C and D. Source: Department of Communicable Diseases and Epidemic Control, Ministry of Health, Ankara, Turkey

Group A Diseases	Group B Diseases	Group C Diseases	Group D Pathogens
AIDS	Smallpox	Acute hemorrhagic fever syndrome	*Campylobacter jejuni*
Acute bloody diarrhea	Epidemic typhus	Creutzfeldt-Jakob disease	*Chlamydia trachomatis* (as a sexually transmitted infection)
Pertussis	Yellow fewer	Echinococcosis	
Brucellosis	Plague	Haemophilus influenzae type B (HiB) meningitis	*Cryptosporidium* ssp.
Diphtheria		Influenza	*Entamoeba histolytica*
Gonorrhea		Leishmaniasis (Kala Azar)	Enterohemorrhagic *E. coli*
HIV		Congenital rubella syndrome	*Giardia intestinalis*
Mumps		Legionnaires' disease	*Listeria monocytogenes*
Rubella		Leprosy	Salmonellosis (Non-typhoidal Salmonellosis)
Measles		Leptospirosis	Shigellosis
Cholera		Subacute sclerosing panencephalitis (SSPE)	
Rabies		Schistosomiasis	
Meningococcal disease		Toxoplasmosis	
Poliomyelitis		Trachoma	
Malaria		Tularemia	
Syphilis			
Anthrax			
Tetanus			
Typhoid fever			
Tuberculosis			
Acute viral hepatitis			
Cutaneous leishmaniasis			
Neonatal tetanus			

collected there do not in practice contribute to overall surveillance. As it can be seen, the surveillance of diseases included in Group C will be a significant experience for the health system of our country. With regard to the specific capacities in relation to these diseases and the provision of diagnostic and treatment services, each health facility at or above the second level will also be obliged to provide notification of these diseases.

Group D, unlike other groups, describes the notification of the "infection agents". This is an important innovation that requires the laboratories to be involved in the direct notification system. The aim here is to obtain information on etiologic agents for those diseases that are still a threat to public health and to be able to carry out epidemiological research when necessary. What is important here is that the laboratory can be a part of the notification system if it has an acceptable diagnostic capacity. Therefore, the Group D surveillance method, together with the indirect role of laboratory on the notification of Groups A, B and C, will bring the dissemination of the work concept based on the standardization and quality assurance.

The Notification System does:

1. Update the list of notifiable infectious diseases
2. Introduce standard case definitions. For example, the case definition for Diphtheriae.
   - Clinical description: An illness characterized by laryngitis, pharyngitis and/or tonsillitis, and adherent membranes of tonsils, pharynx and/or nose (pseudo-membrane).
   - Laboratory criteria for diagnosis: Isolation of toxigenic *Corynebacterium diphtheriae* from a clinical specimen such as pseudomembrane, oropharyngeal or nasal smear.
   - Case classification: (1) Probable case: A case that meets the clinical description. (2) Confirmed case: (a) A probable case that is laboratory confirmed, or (b) A probable case linked epidemiologically to a confirmed case. Note: Persons with positive *C. diphtheriae* cultures who do not meet the clinical description (i.e. asymptomatic carriers) should not be reported as probable or confirmed diphtheria cases. They have to be given only prophylactic treatment and monitored [8].
3. Establish group criteria in the declaration of diseases according to their characteristics. For example, Group A includes diseases which can be easily diagnosed at all levels of health services.
4. Include some new infectious agents in the notification list.
5. Involve direct (Group D, or infectious agents) and indirect participation (Groups A, B, C diseases) of the laboratories within the system.

17.4 Preparation for Medical Response

The intentional use of biological agents is very difficult to anticipate. The release and spread of a contagious agent, such as the smallpox virus, could prove catastrophic if measures for control were not promptly and effectively applied.

A biological crisis may involve many factors, such as location of the attack, population, characteristics of biological agent, treatment and prophylaxis capabilities, and environmental conditions. All these factors must be considered, and given that any such attack is a criminal act, a thorough investigation must also be performed, which may include local, regional, or national authorities. Forensic microbiology is a multidisciplinary field of science which aims to establish the pathogen involved in an outbreak and its source with the ultimate goal of securing the prosecution of the guilty party [3].

Successful preparation will depend upon the development of a well-orchestrated plan to be used by first responders for bioterrorism. They will be epidemiologist, infectious diseases experts and intensive care specialists.

The response strategies to bioterrorism must be continuously improved, in parallel with development of a real time surveillance system, to provide enhanced capabilities for the identification of the biological agent, and the most effective prophylaxis measures and treatment.

Funds are being made available to strengthen the public health and medical infrastructure: smallpox vaccines, antibiotics and other products have been stockpiled; a national network of diagnostic laboratories has been created; and biodefence research programmes are now underway.

It is clear, however, that preventing proliferation and use of biological weapons will be extremely difficult. The "recipes" for making biological weapons have been available on the Internet for many years, and even groups with modest finances and basic training in biology and bioengineering could develop an effective weapon at a minimal cost. Detection of those intending to use biological weapons is next to impossible. In reality, the first evidence of a biological attack will very likely be the appearance of cases in hospital emergency rooms. The rapidity with which those manning emergency rooms and others, such as infectious disease specialists and laboratory scientists, are able to reach a proper diagnosis in addition to the speed with which preventative and therapeutic measures are applied could well determine the difference between thousands and, perhaps, tens of thousands of casualties. Indeed, the destiny of the health staff is depending on their own performance in dealing with a crisis.

However, few of them will have ever seen patients with diseases caused by those agents most likely to be employed, namely smallpox, plague or anthrax. It is therefore essential that front line healthcare providers are properly trained so that the laboratory staff, clinician, or nurse who sees the first patient or wave of patients can recognize the danger early and sound the alarm [10]. In addition, biodefence system must be reinforced in order to ensure a rapid, efficient response in the event of another biological attack. Such measures would include:

1. Improved communications and information dissemination,
2. Increased laboratory capacity,
3. Improved surveillance, detection, and diagnosis,
4. Strengthened response at the local level.

17.5 Bioterrorism and Preparedness in Turkey

Turkey's geo-strategic location elevates its risk in terms of bioterrorism and, given the principle of "every country should establish its own health planning and organization depending on its own conditions", a superior bioterrorism defence organization is urgently needed [6].

The counteraction of chemical and biological threats is the responsibility of the Prime Minister. The Ministry of Defence, Ministry of Health, Turkish Armed Forces, Ministry of the Interior, and local authorities are the other important components of the entire defence system. In the case of any CBRN attack, the Disaster and Emergency Management Presidency (DEMP) is responsible for the whole medical defence system of Turkey. DEMP was tasked as the leading body with the management of chemical, biological, radiological, and nuclear (CBRN) hazards on 3 May 2012 as well as coordinating national CBRN risk analysis with other stakeholders (Governorships, General Staff, Turkish Atomic Energy Authority, and Ministries of Science Industry and Technology, of Environment and Urban Development, of Foreign Affairs, of Food, Agriculture, and Livestock, of Customs and Trade, of Internal Affairs, of Forestry and Water Management, and of Health). The detailed roles and responsibilities were also determined with the regulation.

The police, governorship, coast guard, and gendarmerie work under control of Ministry of the Interior. In the regions, the most effective institutions are the Directorate of Health and hospitals under control of the Ministry of Health. Most of the hospitals play a key role in the event of bio-attacks. Civilian and military authorities work in close coordination in peace time.

By law, in peripheral regions, the regional civilian defence teams of hospitals and the police department work under the control of the Governor. As is the case in most countries, the Turkish Armed Forces have some special facilities and in the case of an unusual epidemiological event, it works under the control of the Governor in coordination with the Turkish General Staff.

17.6 Civilian Defence Organization

Two consecutive major earthquakes in 1999 triggered a turning point in disaster management in Turkey as pre-disaster measures came onto the agenda of the government and the country. Prior to these earthquakes, Turkey's disaster management system was mainly focused on the post-disaster period and there was no incentive or legislation to encourage risk analysis or risk reduction approaches. Both academic and technical authorities agreed that there was an overwhelming need for the country to develop pre-disaster measures involving legislative revision and administrative restructuring.

According to Act No. 5902, "Establishment of Disaster and Emergency Management Presidency", dated 29 May 2009, the following bodies were closed:

1. General Directorate of Turkish Emergency Management under Prime Ministry,
2. General Directorate of Civil Defence under Ministry of Interior,
3. General Directorate of Disaster Affairs under Ministry of Public Works and Settlement.

As stipulated in the act, the duties of these institutions became unified under a single independent authority called "Disaster and Emergency Management Presidency" (DEMP).

In order to ensure the necessary measures are taken to deal with emergency management and civil protection issues nationwide, the presidency conducts pre-incident works, such as preparedness, mitigation and risk management, mid-incident works such as response, and post-incident works such as recovery and reconstruction.

Among the governmental, non-governmental (NGOs) and private institutions, DEMP provides coordination and formulates and implements policies.

The Working Group for Biological Warning of CBRN weapons and related organizations is subordinated to the Department of Civil Defence and is responsible for making preparations and organizing the response to biological weapons. Other components of the Civil Defence Unit are the Working Group of Civil Defence Planning, the Working Group of Mobilization and the Working Group of Civil Defence Training and Foreign Relations.

Duties of the Civil Defence Department:

1. To plan, carry out and supervise civil defence services in governmental and private institutions/organizations,
2. To plan and conduct activities for non-armed protection, rescue, emergency rescue and first-aid,
3. To determine the civilian resources that would be needed during mobilization and war,
4. To work to get the support of the public for civil defence efforts and to maintain good public morale,
5. To determine the measures to be taken to counter chemical, biological, nuclear and radiological threats and hazards and to ensure coordination between ministries, and governmental and private institutions/agencies to achieve this aim.

17.7 The Role of the Ministry of Health

Medical countermeasures on the civilian side are taken by the Ministry of Health through hospitals and the health directorate of governorships. In every province, one hospital is chosen to specialize in biological defence. Although other hospitals have some preparedness against a biological event, this one has drugs (for active/passive prophylaxis, treatment and rehabilitation) and personnel (doctors, nurses, paramedics, laboratory technicians and other auxiliary staff) well-versed in the field of biological defence. Different programmes are applied under the direction of the Ministry of Health: planning and administration; the training of private institutions and laboratories; response; and the creation of health CBRN policy. Funds for the development of these programmes were assigned to the MoH. Countering Weapons of Mass Destruction and Personal Protection Training is a course for trainers, which has been available since 2001. Training activities within the specific disciplines are given, and special training and conferences are organized for the police, fire department, and government agencies.

Health and civil defence workers, fire fighters, the police force, municipality personnel and the Turkish Armed Forces organize joint exercises. In addition, local health units work together with the first intervention teams.

Currently, there are no BSL-4 laboratories in Turkey, but the number of BSL-3 labs is to be increased to assist in the detection of biological agents across the country.

17.8 Military Medical Organizations

The Turkish Armed Forces have their own organization that deals with biological and chemical events. At the operational level, CBRN detection, identification, monitoring, warning, and reporting are executed by land forces, the air force and navy under the control of General Staff, which aims to ensure close coordination between these headquarters. However, medical countermeasures are taken by TAF MEDCOM.

The institutions that execute the biological defence of headquarters are: the Turkish Armed Forces CBRN Defence School and CBRN Defence Battalion (all headquarters), Yildizlar Education Center (Navy), CBRN defence teams and EOD/EOR Teams (Navy and Air Forces) These units have both educational and operational tasks.

Military medical countermeasures against bioterrorism are taken by TAF MEDCOM through the Gulhane Military Medical Academy, military hospitals, infirmaries and dispensaries. The first level of biological defence activities is made by infirmaries and dispensaries in TAF. In the case of a biological event, these facilities respond and this includes medical treatment to some extent. They subsequently evacuate the casualties to military hospitals. The second and third level activities are performed by the Military Medical Academy and military hospitals. In the medical academy, the Department of Medical CBRN Defence Council coordinates all defensive activities, and some related departments. These related departments are: the Department of Medical CBRN Defence, the Department of Microbiology, the Department of Biochemistry, the Department of Infectious Diseases, the Department of Toxicology, the Center of Pharmaceutical Sciences, the Department of Emergency Medicine, all of which help the Department of Medical CBRN Defence Council conduct its defensive activities. Other activities of medical defence against biological events are laboratory activities, academic and administrative activities, research and development, the training of CBRN medical first-aid and rescue teams, and the education of medical staff, which are conducted by the Medical CBRN Defence Council. In addition, the "CBRN Medical First Aid and Rescue Team" is an operational unit that is a component of defence capacity of the academy which, in the situation of a biological attack in a military area or during any operation on a battlefield, would spring in action in accordance with its task definition and ability. The team consists of doctors, non-commissioned officers, nurses and civil servants. The preparedness and organization level of the hospital has a vital importance in terms of reducing the damaging effects of a biological attack. To this end, in military hospitals, a defence organization model is applied for biological attack.

The execution of the system is the responsibility of a "coordinator". The coordinator is a doctor chosen by the head physician. The Defence Council consists of specialist physicians and other health care providers who are experienced in medical chem-bio defence. The council helps the coordinator in the execution of their duties and works under their control. "The First Aid and Rescue Team" is a key element of the defence organization and works under the control of the coordinator [11].

17.9 Conclusion

Turkey is ready for a possible bioterrorist attack and this level of preparedness will only increase as time passes, and even though the current perception of risk is considered to be low, in a rapidly changing world, being ready is the prudent choice given that those perceptions can change at any time.

References

1. Christopher GW, Cieslak TJ, Pavlin JA, Eitzen EM (1997) Biological warfare. A historical perspective. JAMA 278:412–417
2. Christopher GW, Cieslak TJ, Pavlin JA, Eitzen EM Jr (1997) Biological warfare: a historical perspective. In: Knobler SL, Mahmoud AAF, Pray LA (eds) Biological threats and terrorism. National Academy Press, Washington, DC
3. Cummings CA, Relman DA (2002) Microbial forensics – cross-examining pathogens. Science 296:1976–1977
4. Cybulski RJ Jr, Sanz P, O'Brien AD (2009) Anthrax vaccination strategies. Mol Aspects Med 30:490–502
5. Demetrius J, Porche DNS RN, CS, FNP (2002) Biological and chemical bioterrorism agents. J Assoc Nurses AIDS Care 13(5):57–64
6. Eren N (2000) Introduction to health management. Somgur Publishing, Ankara
7. Meselson M, Guillemin J, Hugh-Jones M, Langmuir A, Popova I, Shelokov A, Yampolskaya O (1994) The Sverdlovsk anthrax outbreak of 1979. Science 266:1202–1208
8. The Ministry of Health Turkey (2003) Field Guide for the Control of Diphtheria, Aydogdu Offset Press, Ankara
9. Mughal MA (2002) Biological terrorism: practical response strategies. CML Army Chemical Review. http://findarticles.com/p/articles/mi_m0IUN/is_2002_July/ai_9196 7980/. Accessed 21 Jun 2011
10. Paul F (2009) Strategies of preparedness response to biological warfare and bioterrorism threats. Springer, Dordrecht
11. Yaren H, Kenar L, Karayilanoglu T (2009) Preparedness against chemical and biological terrorism in turkey and civilian-army collaboration. In: Dishowsky C, Pivovarow A (eds) New approaches in counteraction to chemical and biological terrorism. Springer, Dordrecht

Chapter 18
Case Study – United States of America

Lisa D. Rotz and Marcelle Layton

Abstract The United States (US) considers the intentional use of a biological agent a serious national security threat. Over the last decade, federal, state, and local governments in the US have made concerted efforts to enhance preparedness within the public health, medical, and emergency response systems to address this threat. These activities span a wide range of areas from the enactment of new legal authorities and legislative changes to significant financial investments to enhance multiple detection and response system capabilities and the adoption of a national command and control structure for response. Many of these investments, although prompted by the concern for bioterrorism, have served to strengthen public health, medical, and emergency response systems overall and have proven invaluable in responses to other large-scale emergencies, such as the 2009 H1N1 influenza pandemic.

18.1 Public Health Infectious Disease Threats

Infectious diseases still account for a significant portion of public health activities in the United States, whether it is monitoring for and responding to foodborne related outbreaks, addressing increases in nosocomial or antibiotic resistant infections, or tackling new and emerging world-wide infectious threats such as Severe Acute Respiratory Syndrome (SARS) or pandemic influenza. Indeed, infectious diseases still account for two of the ten leading causes of death in the United States [5].

L.D. Rotz (✉)
Centers For Disease Control and Prevention (CDC), Atlanta, GA, USA
e-mail: lrotz@cdc.gov

M. Layton
New York City Department of Health and Mental Hygiene, New York, NY, USA
e-mail: mlayton@health.nyc.gov

I. Hunger et al. (eds.), *Biopreparedness and Public Health: Exploring Synergies*, NATO Science for Peace and Security Series A: Chemistry and Biology,
DOI 10.1007/978-94-007-5273-3_18,

The intentional use of a biological agent is also something that the United States considers a serious threat and the federal, state, and local governments in the US have made concerted efforts to enhance preparedness and capabilities within the public health, medical, and emergency response systems to address this threat. In 2001, this concern became a reality for the US when several letters containing anthrax spores were sent through the postal system to individuals and organizations [14]. This resulted in 22 cases of anthrax (11 inhalational and 11 cutaneous) with five deaths. Although this event may not have been the type of "mass-casualty" situation most bioterrorism preparedness planning activities were targeting, it still resulted in significant response efforts and cost; over 10,000 individuals were offered antibiotic prophylaxis because of possible exposures, over one million clinical and environmental specimens were tested, and hundreds of millions of dollars were spent on decontamination of the buildings where the letters were processed or opened [12, 22].

Although many infectious agents are capable of causing human illness, some are much more capable of causing significant morbidity and mortality if successfully used as a bioterrorism agent. In 2000, the Centers for Disease Control and Prevention (CDC) developed a process to prioritize biological threat agents based on evaluation of the following threat agent characteristics: (1) public health impact from ability to cause illness or death, (2) ability to be produced and delivered in a way that could expose a large number of people, (3) existing public perceptions of a biological agent that could contribute to heightened fear and panic, and (4) requires significant special preparedness efforts in order to diagnose, treat, or prevent illness [20]. Based on these characteristics, biological threat agents were prioritized into three different tiers. Category A (highest threat tier) included *Bacillus anthracis* (anthrax), Variola virus (smallpox), *Yersinia pestis* (plague), *Francisella tularensis* (tularemia), Clostridium botulinum toxin (botulism), and the Filo and Arenaviruses (e.g., Ebola and Marburg virus) that cause viral hemorrhagic fevers. Category B and C were lower threat tiers and included agents such as *Burkholderia mallei* and *B. pseudomallei*, *Rickettsia prowasekii* (Category B), and emerging threats such as Nipah virus (Category C). Following the release of Homeland Security Presidential Directive 10 (HSPD-10) in April 2004, the US Department of Homeland Security (DHS) became responsible for issuing biannual assessments of biological threats in order to guide the prioritization of ongoing investments in research, development, planning, and preparedness [23].

18.2 Preparedness for Public Health Emergencies

The United States has made significant investments in terrorism preparedness and response coordination over the last two decades that includes the implementation of new policies, legislation, and legal authorities in addition to significant funding investments. In 1995, Presidential Directive 39 added a terrorism annex to the Federal Response plan and defined responsibilities of federal agencies in responding to terrorism [25]. The Homeland Security Act of 2002 established the Department of Homeland Security (DHS), a new cabinet level office whose primary mission is to prevent or reduce vulnerability of the United States to terrorism at home; coordinate homeland security responsibilities between the federal government and state, local and private entities; and minimize damage resulting from attacks and assist in the recovery. In 2003, Homeland Security Presidential Directive 5 (HSPD-5) established a nationwide system to coordinate responses to emergencies between local, state, and federal governments and responding organizations and to administer this all hazards National Response Plan through a National Incident Management System (NIMS) that provides for unified command and better multi-agency coordination [24]. Other Presidential Directives and legislation enacted in the US since the World Trade Center and anthrax letter events in 2001 have provided stronger legal frameworks and public health capacity to prevent, prepare, and respond to intentional acts of biological terrorism. The 2002 Public Health Security and Bioterrorism Preparedness Response Act (PHSBPRA) established new requirements for possession, use, and transfer of selected biological agents and toxins (Select Agent List) that could pose threats to human, animal, and plant health and safety as well as established other authorizations and appropriations necessary to carry out essential public health and medical preparedness and response activities [19]. This act authorized more than 1.5 billion US dollars in grants to state and local governments and healthcare facilities to improve planning, training, detection, and response capacity as well as funding to expand the federal Strategic National Stockpile of medications and vaccines and upgrade food inspection capacity and CDC facilities that deal with public health threats. The Project Bioshield Act (July 2004) and Pandemic and All-Hazards Preparedness Act (December 2006) also specifically provided for new authorities and funding to address significant gaps that existed for the development, acquisition, and utilization of medical countermeasures (e.g. antimicrobials, vaccines, chemical antidotes) for chemical, biological, radiological, and nuclear (CBRN) threats.

In 2002, the CDC asked the Center for Law and Public Health at Georgetown and Johns Hopkins Universities to draft a model state public health law (the Model State Emergency Health Powers Act or Model Act) for state and local jurisdictions to use in addressing either bioterrorism or naturally occurring disease outbreaks [9]. The Model Act (available at http://www.publichealthlaw.net/MSEHPA/MSEHPA.pdf) outlines five major public health functions to be allowed by law including preparedness, surveillance, management of property, protection of persons, and communication. In addition to ensuring sufficient authority to collect disease surveillance data, conduct contact tracing, and provide preventive measures to those at risk, public health laws must enable local health officials to implement quarantine measures, if needed, to control a contagious disease outbreak with epidemic potential that could lead to severe morbidity or mortality (e.g. smallpox). This authority should be linked with specific, scientifically appropriate criteria that would be met before quarantine could be implemented. In addition, public health laws should provide for due process measures to protect those affected. Ideally, quarantine strategies would be determined and operational procedures would be in place prior to an emergency.

Ongoing broad-based investments to improve response planning and coordination, surveillance, training, information systems, and communications have been made that serve to improve public health capacity for all threats and hazards. Starting in 1999, the US Government began providing funding to 62 state, local, and territorial health departments to build stronger capacity for surveillance and epidemiology, laboratory diagnostic capacity, communications, countermeasure distribution, and emergency response planning, exercise, and evaluation. The initial investment into these public health system upgrades started at 40 million US dollars per year with a primary focus on addressing bioterrorism threats. Following the events of 2001, funding to support enhancements in the national public health infrastructure increased to approximately 1.5 billion per year. The current state of progress towards specific preparedness goals identified for CDC funded preparedness and response activities in the 62 state, local, and US insular areas is provided in the "2010 Report – Public Health Preparedness: Strengthening the Nation's Emergency Response State by State" which can be found online at http://emergency.cdc.gov/publications/2010phprep/.

Additionally, more targeted investments have been made that address surveillance, detection, and illness prevention or treatment needs for specific high priority threats. Examples of these targeted initiatives include the Laboratory Response Network (LRN), the Strategic National Stockpile (SNS), and an environmental monitoring system called BioWatch. In 1999, the CDC and other partners formed the Laboratory Response Network (LRN) [3]. The LRN is a network of approximately 170 national and international public health, veterinary, agriculture, food, military, and environmental laboratories that have increased diagnostic capability for the rapid identification of multiple biological and chemical threat agents in multiple sample types. Participation in the network is voluntary and these pre-existing laboratories work under a single operational plan and adhere to policies on safety, security, and bio-containment. LRN members agree to perform testing using LRN procedures and are provided training, equipment, rapid detection assays and reagents, protocols, and secured communication and data reporting systems to increase testing and laboratory response capabilities in a standardized and coordinated fashion. There are three types of laboratory designation within the LRN: national, reference, and sentinel. National labs have unique capabilities and resources that allow them to handle highly infectious agents and perform strain-level identification and other agent characterization testing. Reference laboratories are mostly based at state and large city health departments and have the capability to perform rapid confirmatory testing for certain agents and toxins while sentinel laboratories (primarily hospital and commercial clinical laboratories) can perform routine clinical testing on patient specimens with additional training and protocols for notification and rapid referral of isolates in the event that they are unable to rule-out a biothreat agent. In addition to the central role the LRN played in detecting and responding to the 2001 anthrax letter event, the commitment to infrastructure support and standardized platform testing capacity within the LRN has also proven extremely beneficial in assisting with more rapid and broader deployment of tests developed in response to other emerging public health threats such as the 2003 Severe Acute

Respiratory Syndrome (SARS) and the 2009 H1N1 avian influenza pandemic. LRN laboratories are also trained on chain-of-custody requirements and protocols which allow them to serve as a local testing resource for law enforcement linked samples where there is a concern for biological threat agents. Approximately 90% of the US population lives within 100 miles of an LRN laboratory, which provides for more rapid access to confirmatory diagnostic testing to evaluate potential illness from or exposures to threat agents.

The SNS (formerly the National Pharmaceutical Stockpile) program began in 1999 to acquire and store a stockpile of medications, vaccines, and other medical supplies whose rapid availability is vitally important for response to a large-scale event involving certain biological, chemical, or radiological agents [4]. Without a pre-purchased and stored stockpile, most of these medications and vaccines would not be readily available through other sources in appropriate amounts or in a timeframe that would allow for the prevention or effective treatment of illness. Partnerships with storage and transportation companies have been created that provide strategically located storage facilities, allowing rapid delivery of SNS materiel to any location in the US or its territories within 12 h of the federal decision to deploy. Certain medical countermeasures may be eligible for the shelf-life extension program managed by the Food and Drug Administration and the Department of Defense, which allows for expiration date extension based on potency and other test results. In addition, agreements with pharmaceutical companies and medication distribution partners have allowed for rotation of certain medications back into the commercial supply chain for use prior to their expiration in order to help mitigate replacement costs. Although the SNS was originally developed as a medical countermeasure response resource for intentional biological, chemical, and radiological emergencies, it has been deployed and used multiple times to support the medical needs of other public health emergencies, including Hurricanes Katrina and Rita, the recent H1N1 influenza pandemic, the 2001 World Trade Center and the anthrax letter attacks.

The successful distribution of the SNS is dependent on the capacity of state and local jurisdictions to rapidly dispense these countermeasures to the public. Planning for the timely provision of antibiotics and/or vaccines to large populations requires the involvement of public health, emergency management, and the local medical community. Mass prophylaxis plans need to consider the specific challenges of potentially vulnerable populations, such as children, pregnant women, and those who are isolated and without resources and social supports, such as the homeless and homebound. Contingency plans for setting up community-based Points of Dispensing (PODs) for mass prophylaxis have been developed by most state and local jurisdictions, with a focus on ensuring sufficient staffing resources, equipment and space requirements, and expediting patient flow. The capacity of health officials to rapidly vaccinate the community was recently tested in the United States during the 2009 H1N1 pandemic and demonstrated the need for flexibility and coordination in distribution of vaccine, including school-based programs, community health centers, pharmacies, and large health department sponsored vaccination clinics.

Multiple initiatives have been supported to further strengthen public health disease surveillance and reporting that include an emphasis on traditional disease reporting as well as the utilization of non-traditional data that may provide an earlier indication of community health events or more likely assist with situational awareness assessments during an identified event [8]. Traditional public health surveillance for illness associated with potential bioterrorism agents relies on enhancing the medical and laboratory communities' familiarity with these agents, with the goal of improved reporting of suspected or confirmed illnesses, as well as reporting of unusual disease manifestations or illness clusters. Most local and state health codes require that physicians, hospitals, and laboratories report a defined list of notifiable infectious diseases. State public health agencies have added CDC Category A and B agents to their reportable disease lists. These lists are available at http://www.cste.org/dnn/Programs andActivities/PublicHealthInformatics/PHIStateReportableWebsites/tabid/1 36/Default.aspx. In addition, recognizing the need to detect newly emergent diseases that are not yet listed on the health code, most states also require reporting of any unusual disease clusters or manifestations. Early recognition of a bioterrorism-associated event depends in large part on astute clinicians and laboratorians recognizing one of the index cases based on a suspicious clinical, radiologic, or laboratory presentation (e.g. a febrile illness associated with chest discomfort and a widened mediastinum on chest radiograph in an otherwise healthy adult suggests inhalation anthrax). Isolated cases presenting at separate hospitals will not be recognized as a potential outbreak unless they are reported promptly to the local health department, where the population-based aberrations in disease trends are more likely to be noticed. Previous examples of astute clinicians recognizing and reporting unusual disease clusters or manifestations that led to the detection of a more widespread outbreak include an outbreak of hantavirus in the southwestern US [7], Legionnaires' disease associated with the whirlpool on a cruise ship [13], an outbreak of *Cyclospora* associated with contaminated raspberries imported from Guatemala [11], and the initial outbreak of West Nile virus in New York City in 1999 [18]. Similarly, the initial detection of anthrax in 2001 was due to a physician who recognized that large gram-positive rods in a patient's cerebrospinal fluid could be *B. anthracis* [1]. By reporting this suspected case of meningeal anthrax, rapid confirmation was facilitated in a state public health LRN reference laboratory. Weeks later, a suspected case of inhalation anthrax was recognized and promptly reported to and confirmed by public health authorities in New York City [17].

With the continued emergence of new zoonotic disease threats, including those related to bioterrorism, local, state, and federal public health agencies have taken steps to improve communication between human and animal health communities. Notifiable disease requirements have been expanded to include reporting by animal health specialists of suspected or confirmed illness in an animal that might be caused by a potential biothreat agent.

Because many medical providers and laboratorians in the United States have limited experience with most potential bioterrorist agents, early diagnosis may be delayed. Therefore, the first indication that a large-scale bioterrorist attack has taken place might be an increase in nonspecific symptoms at the community level. Surveillance for these increases in nonspecific syndromes (e.g. respiratory, gastrointestinal, or neurologic) constitutes the cornerstone of syndromic surveillance used for emergency response purposes.

Many health jurisdictions have begun collecting and monitoring other types of health-related information such as symptom complexes presented during emergency room visits (e.g. lower respiratory tract illness, gastrointestinal illness, rash with fever), healthcare utilization information (e.g. emergency room visits, 911 calls), or other data that may be affected by a community-wide health event (e.g. school absenteeism, flu or diarrhea over-the-counter medication sales) [10, 15].

Though the approaches and cost for implementing syndromic surveillance vary, the tools and concepts for syndromic surveillance are adaptable and have been successfully implemented in both developed and developing countries to address routine surveillance, outbreak monitoring, and health security needs [6]. While initially conceived for early detection for bioterrorism, these systems also can be used to monitor natural infectious disease outbreaks and trends in noninfectious events of public health importance. Information from syndromic systems has proven to be useful for detecting, monitoring, and characterizing seasonal outbreaks of influenza, winter gastroenteritis (e.g. norovirus and rotavirus) and asthma. Furthermore, syndromic systems were utilized extensively in the US during the novel H1N1 influenza pandemic of 2009, along with other methods, to estimate the scale of community-wide influenza transmission.

An additional concept to specifically improve early detection of an intentional biological agent release is the use of environmental monitoring systems. If an agent can be detected quickly following an aerosol release, response timelines can be significantly improved, allowing for more time to intervene and potentially prevent illness in a significant portion of the exposed population. In 2003, the United States implemented BioWatch, an environmental monitoring system that consists of a network of samplers that collect air on a continuing cycle [21]. Filters from the monitors are removed on a frequent basis and screened in a laboratory for the presence of several biological threat agents. BioWatch is currently operational in multiple US cities. Environmental monitoring in this fashion requires a significant financial commitment and is a complex system to operate as experience with this type of system was limited prior to its implementation. Natural environmental presence of the target organisms and/or very closely related organisms and the size of the area to be monitored present ongoing challenges for establishing system sensitivities and specificities that appropriately balance the potential value of early detection of a bioterrorism attack with the risk of inappropriately responding to a positive test that is caused by naturally occurring organisms in the environment. A separate system of detectors has also been deployed that monitors the US mail system, the method of "dissemination" used in the 2001 anthrax letter attacks. The US Postal BioHazard Detection System (BDS) has been operational since 2004 [16]. Unlike traditional disease and syndromic surveillance systems for human and animal health which monitor for both intentional and naturally occurring disease, these environmental systems are single purpose with the primary focus being early warning of bioterrorism.

One of the more effective preparedness planning tools are tabletop and field exercises, with involvement of representatives from key local, state, and federal agencies, as well as representatives from the local medical and laboratory communities.

These exercises provide the opportunity to test assumptions in existing plans, and work out issues related to decision-making authority and respective roles and responsibilities among the various disciplines that would be involved in responding to a bioterrorist attack or other local emergency. Post exercise debriefings should be conducted to highlight gaps in preparedness that can then be addressed through follow-up planning meetings and revision of written plans, if indicated, and re-evaluated with repeat exercises.

18.3 Response to Public Health Emergencies

Depending upon the size and scope, responses to public health emergencies may involve resources and responsibilities that span multiple agencies at the local (city or county), state, and federal government levels. Emergency events begin at the community level (single or multiple communities) and local personnel and resources (medical, public health, emergency services, police, fire, etc.) provide the initial response. If local resources are overwhelmed or authorities require special assistance or resources that are not locally available, assistance from the state or federal level can be requested. This may be done through a direct assistance request to an agency or agencies (e.g. a request to CDC to assist with a food outbreak investigation or test samples) or through the formal declaration of an emergency that activates state and federal emergency support functions (e.g. declaration of state of emergency that activates the Federal Emergency Management Agency (FEMA) and other federal assistance as needed through the National Response Framework (NRF) and the associated Emergency Support Functions (ESF)). Emergency responses and their coordination in the US primarily involve civilian agencies and authorities, with the military providing support as needed.

Central to the ability to successfully coordinate a response to a large-scale emergency is the ability to integrate information flow, resources, and personnel into an organizational structure that is similar across all responding agencies, whether the emergency is primarily public health in nature or due to some other cause. This Incident Management System or Incident Command System (ICS) structure, has been used for many years by traditional first responder agencies such as fire and law enforcement and was formally identified as the national emergency response structure in 2003 [24]. ICS has also been adopted and used to a much greater extent by federal, state, and local public health agencies responding to public health emergencies. CDC utilized the ICS to coordinate its response to public health emergencies such as the 2009 H1N1 pandemic and multi-state foodborne outbreaks but has also benefited from better integration of its response activities into larger-scale, multi-hazard emergency responses such as Hurricane Katrina and the recent Haiti earthquake.

The US Department of Health and Human Services (DHHS) has the lead for coordinating the federal public health and medical services support functions outlined in ESF 8 (http://www.fema.gov/pdf/emergency/nrf/nrf-esf-08.pdf).

These support functions include response activities in the following areas: (1) assessment of public health/medical needs, (2) health surveillance, (3) medical care personnel, (4) health/medical/veterinary equipment and supplies, (5) patient evacuation, (6) patient care, (7) safety and security of drugs, biologics, and medical devices, (8) blood and blood products, (9) food safety and security, (10) agriculture safety and security, (11) all-hazard public health and medical consultation, technical assistance, and support, (12) behavioral health care, (13) public health and medical information, (14) vector control, (15) potable water/wastewater and solid waste disposal, (16) mass fatality management, victim identification, and decontaminating remains, and (17) veterinary medical support. Several agencies exist within DHHS that help carry out these activities, including CDC, the Food and Drug Administration (FDA), the National Institutes for Health (NIH), and the Substance Abuse and Mental Health Services Administration (SAMHSA) among others. In addition, DHHS manages the National Disaster Medical System (NDMS) which includes disaster medical, surgical, and mortuary response teams as well as veterinary response teams. In addition to providing medical response to a disaster area, NDMS also coordinates patient movement into hospital care in unaffected areas for definitive medical care with the support of the Department of Defense (DoD). In addition to DoD, multiple other agencies and departments provide support to DHHS for ESF8 functions, including the Department of Agriculture (DoA), DHS, FEMA, the Department of Transportation (DoT), the Department of Veterans Affairs (VA), the American Red Cross (ARC), and others.

Once a bioterrorist event is recognized and then confirmed by laboratory testing, there will be a need for large-scale mobilization of surveillance and epidemiologic investigations. The focus of these investigations will be (1) tracking the number of cases to define the scope of the incident and (2) performing epidemiologic investigations to determine the common source(s) and site(s) of exposure. This information will be most critical in the event of a covert bioterrorist event to determine where and when the attack occurred, and who else may have been potentially exposed (either at the event or due to downwind distribution of the aerosol) and thus require prophylaxis. As active surveillance would need to be initiated rapidly once a bioterrorist event is recognized, many local and state health departments have developed materials and plans to facilitate the ability to rapidly implement an investigation, including template surveillance instruments and protocols for urgently mobilizing and deploying active surveillance surge teams to hospitals in the affected area.

Response to public health emergencies that result from an intentional biothreat agent, such as the 2001 US anthrax letter attacks, have an added investigational and coordination complexity due to the necessary law enforcement component of the event [2]. If an event is known to be secondary to an intentional act, local law enforcement officials and the Federal Bureau of Investigation (FBI) have a greater leadership role in coordinating the investigation and communication, however, public health and other responding entities are still responsible for carrying out their usual surveillance and emergency response activities. In this scenario, activities such as interviewing victims to determine the common site and/or sources of exposure, specimen or sample collection and testing, and public messaging would be coordinated with the FBI or other law enforcement officials in order to preserve evidence and investigative information that may be essential for attribution and conviction of the perpetrators. Some activities such as sample collection or victim interviews may even need to be planned and conducted jointly by public health and law enforcement officials. Although law enforcement has the responsibility for conducting the criminal investigation, their primary mission is also the preservation of life and health and investigative activities are targeted towards accomplishing that goal in addition to obtaining the evidence needed to identify and convict those responsible. Many local, state, and federal public health and law enforcement authorities in the US have recognized the investigation and communication coordination that would be required in a bioterrorism or other intentional chemical, radiological, or toxin induced event that affects the health of individuals or communities and have established working relationships for preparedness as well as formalized agreements for information sharing and joint investigative activities in this type of event. A model for a Memorandum of Understanding (MOU) that can be used to create formalized working agreements between public health and law enforcement officials was developed by a working group convened by the CDC and the US Department of Justice. This model MOU has been distributed to state and local authorities and a copy can be requested through the CDC Public Health Law Practice website at http://www2a.cdc.gov/phlp/mounote.asp.

18.4 Summary

The United States considers bioterrorism a serious threat to its national security and has made concerted efforts over the last decade to bolster public health and other response capacity capabilities. Many of these efforts, though initially begun to address the needs for bioterrorism preparedness, have proven beneficial for public health in responding to other emergencies, including those due to naturally occurring disease threats such as pandemic influenza. Specifically, efforts that focused on improving: (1) laboratory diagnostic capacity, (2) surveillance data sources, analysis, and reporting, (3) risk communication (4) emergency response planning and training, and (5) overall response coordination have proven extremely beneficial for supporting public health responses to all types of health threats. In most state and local health departments in the US, bioterrorism surveillance and response capacity is fully integrated into the general infectious disease and all hazards emergency response infrastructure. The same staff that surveil for and respond to both routine and emergency infectious disease outbreaks would be called upon to respond to a bioterrorism attack. This dual-use capacity is more efficient and ensures that front line public health staff maintain and exercise the skills required to detect and respond to disease threats, regardless of whether intentional or natural. The 2009 H1N1 pandemic provided one of the best training opportunities for what might be encountered in the event of a large scale bioterrorist outbreak, including the need to implement enhanced surveillance to provide greater real time situational awareness, with the initial reliance on the public health laboratory system for reference testing, and the implementation of a large scale vaccination campaign. Although bioterrorism is not accorded the same level of concern everywhere, investments that help build or support stronger public health and medical systems provide the foundation for responding to all health threats and are essential, should an unthinkable event such as a large-scale bioterrorism attack occur.

References

1. Bush LM, Abrams BH, Johnson CC (2001) Index case of fatal inhalational anthrax due to bioterrorism in the United States. N Engl J Med 1(345):1607–1610
2. Butler JC, Cohen ML, Friedman CR, Scripp RM, Watz CG (2002) Collaboration between public health and law enforcement: new paradigms and partnerships for bioterrorism planning and response. Emerg Infect Dis 8(10). http://www.cdc.gov/ncidod/ EID/vol8no10/02-0400.htm . Accessed 4 Apr 2011
3. CDC (1999a) Emergency preparedness and response: the laboratory response network partners in preparedness. http://emergency.cdc.gov/lrn/. Accessed 8 Mar 2011
4. CDC (1999b) Emergency preparedness and response: strategic national stockpile, http://www.cdc.gov/phpr/stockpile.htm. Accessed 8 Mar 2011
5. CDC (2007) Leading causes of death. http://www.cdc.gov/nchs/FASTATS/lcod.htm. Accessed 4 Apr 2011
6. Chretien J, Burkom HS, Sedyaningsih ER, Larasati RP, Lescano AG et al (2008) Syndromic surveillance: adapting innovations to developing settings. PLoS Med 5(3):e72, doi:10.1371/journal.pmed.0050072. http://www.plosmedicine.org/article/ info%3Adoi%2 F10.1371%2Fjournal.pmed.0050072. Accessed 4 Apr 2011
7. Duchin JS, Koster FT, Peters CJ et al (1994) Hantavirus pulmonary syndrome: a clinical description of 17 patients with a newly recognized disease. N Engl J Med 330(14):949–955
8. Fricker RD Jr (2008) Syndromic surveillance. In: Melnick E, Everitt B (eds) Encyclopedia of quantitative risk analysis and assessment. Wiley, Chichester, pp 1743–1752, Hoboken, NJ. http://www.wiley.com/WileyCDA/
9. Gostin LO, Sapsin JW, Teret SP, Burris S, Mair JS, Hodge JG Jr, Vernick JS (2002) The model state emergency health powers act: planning for and response to bioterrorism and naturally occurring infectious diseases. JAMA 288(5):622–628
10. Henning KJ (2004) Overview of syndromic surveillance: what is syndromic surveillance. Morb Mortal Wkly Rep 53(suppl):5–11. http://www.cdc.gov/mmwr/ preview/mmwrhtml/su5301a3.htm. Accessed 8 Mar 2011
11. Herwaldt BL, Ackers M, Cyclospora Working Group (1997) An outbreak in 1996 of cyclosporiasis associated with imported raspberries. N Engl J Med 336(22):1548–1556
12. Hughes JM, Gerberding JL (2002) Anthrax bioterrorism: lessons learned and future directions. Emerging Infectious Diseases 8(10). http://www.cdc.gov/ncidod/EID/ vol8no10/02-0466.htm. Accessed 4 Apr 2011
13. Jernigan DB, Hofmann J, Cetron MS et al (1996) Outbreak of Legionnaires' disease among cruise ship passengers exposed to a contaminated whirlpool spa. Lancet 347(9000):494–499
14. Jernigan DB, Raghunathan PL, Bell BP, Brechner R, Bresnitz EA, Butler JC et al (2002) Investigation of bioterrorism-related anthrax, United States, 2001: epidemiologic findings. Emerging Infectious Diseases 8(10). http://www.cdc.gov/ncidod/EID/ vol8no10/02-0353.htm. Accessed 4 April 2011

15. Mandl KD, Overhage JM, Wagner MM, Lober WB, Sebastiani P, Mostashari F et al (2004) Implementing syndromic surveillance: a practical guide informed by the early experience. J Am Med Inf Assoc 11(2):141–150, doi: 10.1197/jamia.M1356. http://www.ncbi.nlm.nih.gov/pmc/articles/PMC353021/. Accessed 8 Mar 2011
16. Meehan PJ, Rosenstein NE, Gillen M, Meyer RF, Keifer MJ, Deitchman S et al (2004) Responding to detection of aerosolized Bacillus anthracis by autonomous detection systems in the workplace. Morb Mortal Wkly Rep 53(suppl):1–11. http://www.cdc.gov/mmwr/preview/mmwrhtml/rr53e430-2a1.htm. Accessed 8 Mar 2011
17. Mina B, Dym JP, Kuepper F et al (2002) Fatal inhalational anthrax with unknown source of exposure in a 61-year-old woman in New York city. JAMA 287(7):858–862
18. Nash D, Mostashari F, Fine A et al (2001) The outbreak of west Nile virus infection in the New York City area in 1999. N Engl J Med 344(24):1807–1814
19. The Public Health Security and Bioterrorism Preparedness and Response Act (2002) http://thomas.loc.gov/cgi-bin/query/F?c107:1:./temp/~c10776ZsrO:e666. Accessed 28 Feb 2011
20. Rotz LD, Khan AS, Lillibridge SR, Ostroff SM, Hughes JM (2002) Public health assessment of potential biological terrorism agents. Emerg Infect Dis 8(2). http://www.cdc.gov/ncidod/eid/vol8no2/01-0164.htm. Accessed 4 Apr 2011
21. Shea DA, Lister SA (2003) The BioWatch program: Detection of bioterrorism. US Congressional Research Service Report No. RL 32152. http://www.fas.org/sgp/crs/ terror/RL32152.html#n_2_. Accessed 10 Mar 2011
22. Shepard CW, Soriano-Gabarro-Soriano M, Zell ER, Hayslett J, Lukacs S, Goldstein S et al (2002) Antimicrobial postexposure prophylaxis for anthrax: adverse events and adherence. Emerg Infect Dis 8(10). http://www.cdc.gov/ncidod/EID/ vol8no10/02-0349.htm. Accessed 4 Apr 2011
23. US Homeland Security Presidential Directive 10 (2004) HSPD-10: Biodefense for the 21st century. www.fas.org/irp/offdocs/nspd/hspd-10.html. Accessed 28 Feb 2011
24. US Homeland Security Presidential Directive 5 (2003) HSPD-5: Management of domestic incidents. http://georgewbush-whitehouse.archives.gov/news/releases/2003/02/20030228–9.html. Accessed 28 Feb 2011
25. US Presidential Decision Directive 39 (1995) Terrorism Incident Annex to the Federal Response Plan. http://www.fas.org/irp/offdocs/pdd39_frp.htm. Accessed 28 Feb 2011

Chapter 19
Concluding Remarks

Iris Hunger, Lisa D. Rotz*, Goran Belojevic, and Vladan Radosavljevic

Abstract The case studies collected in this book illustrate the considerable differences in bioterrorism threat perception, levels of biopreparedness, and views on how to balance general public health efforts and biopreparedness measures. While investing too little in biopreparedness leaves countries ill-equipped for a potential disaster, spending too much might create a threat in itself, for example, by redirecting resources away from dealing with everyday health threats. Countries, regardless of perceived threat or economic capacity, should aim to develop and maintain a public health system capable of a well-planned, well-rehearsed, and rapidly executed response to natural health emergencies. Such a system will diminish the consequences of both a naturally occurring health emergency and a bioterrorist attack, should it occur.

---

*The findings and conclusions in this chapter are those of the author and no not necessarily represent the views of the Centers for Disease Control and Prevention.

I. Hunger (✉)
Research Group for Biological Arms Control, Carl Friedrich von Weizsäcker Centre for Science and Peace Research, University of Hamburg, Hamburg, Germany
e-mail: irishunger@versanet.de

L.D. Rotz
Centers for Disease Control and Prevention (CDC), Atlanta, GA, USA
e-mail: lrotz@cdc.gov

G. Belojevic
Institute of Hygiene and Medical Ecology, Faculty of Medicine, University of Belgrade, Belgrade, Serbia
e-mail: goran.belojevic@hotmail.com

V. Radosavljevic
Military Academy, University of Defence, Belgrade, Serbia

Medical Corps Headquarters, Army of Serbia, Belgrade, Serbia
e-mail: vladanr4@gmail.com

I. Hunger et al. (eds.), *Biopreparedness and Public Health: Exploring Synergies*, NATO Science for Peace and Security Series A: Chemistry and Biology,
DOI 10.1007/978-94-007-5273-3_19,

How to balance efforts to improve public health in general with efforts to counter bioterrorism has been a concern of experts at least since the anthrax letter attacks in the USA in 2001. Finding this balance is particularly difficult, because – as the case studies in this book illustrate – the agents of public health concern match agents of bioterrorism concern only to a very limited degree. Even regarding just the agents of bioterrorism concern, there is little agreement about which agent is of high, low, or no concern. An impressive number of agent lists exist in both the public health and counterterrorism areas, sometimes several lists in one country.

Bioterrorism events (excluding hoaxes) are a subset of health emergency events. They are part of the group of unexpected, rare disease events that challenge public health systems globally and continuously. Examples of such unusual disease events are imported cases of dangerous infectious diseases such as a Lassa fever case in Germany in 2000 [3], cases of rare diseases such as anthrax in intravenous drug users in 2009–2010 across Europe [1, 2], the appearance of dangerous new diseases such as SARS in 2003 [4], or cases of known diseases with unfamiliar characteristics such as enterohaemorrhagic *Escherichia coli* O104:H4 infections in Germany in 2011 [5]. None of these were known to be intentionally inflicted. Nevertheless, they were unusual because they concern known diseases that normally do not occur in a country, emerging diseases, or diseases exhibiting new characteristics. Such disease events challenge prevention, detection, diagnostic, and treatment capabilities of public health systems.

Disease outbreaks due to bioterrorism are, from a public health point of view, just one of the challenges facing a public health system, and they will initially be dealt with as natural disease outbreaks would be. Once the deliberate character of the outbreak has been established, a few specific points need to be considered, such as a sudden demand – justified or not – for postexposure prophylaxis, the probability of shortages of specific medical countermeasures, possibly more extensive decontamination requirements and expectations, and an altered communication strategy. From a legal point of view, a bioterrorism event is, of course, a completely different matter than a naturally occurring disease outbreak. The related law enforcement forensic investigations may impact the public health response, but may have similar immediate urgency if there is serious concern about follow-up attacks. Therefore, public health and law enforcement officials must plan and work together to coordinate their investigations to save lives through mitigating the impact to those already exposed (investigation to determine who was exposed and how treatment and/or preventive measures can be implemented), and preventing additional attacks/exposures (by identifying and arresting the perpetrators).

For successfully coping with unusual disease events, a robust public health system is essential. In particular, the sooner an event is recognized, the better. Robust disease surveillance mechanisms are therefore of utmost importance. Rapid access to reliable and accurate medical data is vital. Ideally, disease surveillance systems provide real-time or near-real-time data, aided or generated by widely-available, rapid, and cheap diagnostic tools. All countries considered in this publication have disease surveillance systems in place, although the number and kind of diseases covered on a routine basis differ. One country operates two additional surveillance systems with the exclusive aim of detecting bioterrorist attacks.

The next priority after identifying an event is to manage and if possible reduce the consequences. The consequences of a bioterrorism event or any other disease outbreak can be reduced significantly by rapid and appropriate medical care and implementation of other public health control measures. Almost all countries surveyed in this publication keep stockpiles of some medications. While for financial reasons, it might not be possible to assure availability of agent-specific medical countermeasures and prophylactics for all agents of potential bioterrorism concern, a number of non-agent-specific response mechanisms can also help limit the consequences of an outbreak (communication plans, quarantine regulations or other social distancing measures, distribution of intensive medical care capacities, plans for utilizing other scarce resources, etc.).

The case studies in this publication illustrate that – while no country completely dismisses the threat from bioterrorism – strong differences in risk perception exist, ranging from "very serious threat" via "one of the possible, albeit improbable, catastrophic events" to "intentional release not likely at this time". Accordingly, views differ on the importance of preparedness and countermeasures specifically for bioterrorism events. Important questions in this regard are "How much money and effort are enough?" and "How much might be too much?" The answer to these questions depends not only on the perceived threat and the level of risk acceptance, but also on the general financial situation of a country. If countermeasures against infectious diseases of known likelihood and impact are inadequate, should a country invest in specific countermeasures for other infectious diseases with largely unknown likelihood and impact, or perhaps seek to develop joint assistance agreements with other international partners?

Investing too little money and thought on biopreparedness leaves countries ill-equipped for a potential disaster. However, spending too much might create a threat in itself by diverting resources from dealing with known health threats. Too much biodefence research might also prompt allegations of offensive weapons development under the guise of biodefence, especially if the level of transparency is low. In addition, biodefence research creates experts, knowledge, and materials that are particularly vulnerable to misuse, especially if not managed properly. Effective oversight of biodefence activities and scientists is vital. At the national level, a biosecurity system has to be in place. At the international level, an open and transparent bioscience community and peer-based control are important to prevent biodefence efforts from being misused for hostile purposes. Last, there is the potential danger of turning public health from a humanitarian focus – nationally and internationally – into a security focus, with the resulting changes in priorities.

The case studies in this book illustrate that countries differ to a great extent in public health preparedness for a bioterrorist attack. Whether they are well prepared or still in the process of developing biopreparedness policy, in almost all countries biopreparedness is part of overall health emergency preparedness, with the ministries of interior and health being the responsible agencies. Involvement of military agencies differs greatly. Some countries, particularly in Eastern Europe, have traditionally left bioterrorism-specific detection, diagnosis and response in the military domain, with little involvement of civilian authorities. In other, mostly Western, countries, the military has a supportive role, with civil agencies leading the preparedness and response charge. Finally, in a few countries, the military and civilian authorities share primary response roles.

We see merit in considering the following principles in designing biopreparedness efforts to maximize synergies between those efforts and global public health:

1. Biopreparedness should be part of a nation's public health and emergency preparedness efforts. Biopreparedness efforts should be based primarily in public health institutions with public health funding, not primarily in military or closed security institutions. This is not to suggest that no other civilian, military, or medical agencies should be involved in biopreparedness efforts. The medical care infrastructure is essential for response, and the military can provide valuable expertise, assistance, information, and ressources. The Ministry of Agriculture would be needed for events involving animal and plant security.
2. The focus of biopreparedness efforts should be on what makes sense from a health threat standpoint, regardless of perception of the bioterrorism threat. Strong disease surveillance systems, laboratory diagnostic capacity, health care system planning, risk communications, and response coordination are all capacities that would serve to mitigate the consequences of multiple types of health threats (e.g., natural disasters, influenza pandemics, outbreaks of emerging diseases), including bioterrorism. Several of these capacities are also called for under the International Health Regulations.
3. Three bioterrorism-specific aspects should be considered, even if resources are extremely limited:
    - A designated person or agency should be responsible and familiar with the issue of bioterrorism and how to plan and respond.
    - Arrangements, especially the relationship with law enforcement entities, should be thought through in advance.
    - Public health and medical personnel should receive continuing education and training. At a minimum, they should know what to look for and whom to call if there are indications of unusual disease events.
4. If countries plan to invest in dedicated research and development of countermeasures against rare diseases such as viral hemorrhagic fevers, such research would best be conducted jointly and in cooperation with countries where the diseases in question are present naturally. The results of this research should be available for public health purposes in countries where such diseases are a natural threat.

Countries, regardless of perceived threat or economic capacity, should aim to develop and maintain a public health system capable of a well-planned, well-rehearsed, and rapidly executed response to natural health emergencies. Such a system will diminish the consequences of both a naturally occurring health emergency and a bioterrorist attack, should it occur, and may also contribute to deterring adversaries from pursuing such attacks.

References

1. ECDC (2010) Joint ECDC and EMCDDA threat assessment. Anthrax outbreak among drug users, UK and Germany. Update: 11 February 2010. http://ecdc.europa.eu/en/activities/sciadvice/Documents/2010-02-11-TA_anthrax_IDU_ECDC-EMCDDA.pdf. Accessed 6 Jun 2012
2. ECDC (2011) Annual epidemiological report. Reporting on 2009 surveillance data and 2010 epidemic intelligence data. 2011, pp. 63–64, 215–216. http://ecdc.europa.eu/en/ publications/publications/1111_sur_annual_epidemiological_report_on_communicable_diseases_in_europe.pdf. Accessed 6 Jun 2012
3. Haas WH, Breuer T, Pfaff G, Schmitz H, Köhler P, Asper M, Emmerich P, Drosten C, Gölnitz U, Fleischer K, Günther S (2003) Imported Lassa fever in Germany: surveillance and management of contact persons. Clin Infect Dis 2003(36):1254–1258. http://cid.oxfordjournals.org/content/36/10/1254.full.pdf. Accessed 4 Jun 2012
4. Parashar UD, Anderson LJ (2004) Severe acute respiratory syndrome: review and lessons of the 2003 outbreak. Int J Epidemiol 33(4): 628–634. http://ije.oxfordjournals.org/content/33/4/628.full.pdf+html. Accessed 4 Jun 2012
5. Robert Koch Institute (2011) Final presentation and evaluation of epidemiological findings in the EHEC O104:H4 outbreak. Germany 2011. Robert Koch Institute. September 2011. http://www.rki.de/EN/Home/EHEC_final_report.pdf. Accessed 4 Jun 2012